SURVIVAL MANUAL FOR NURSING STUDENTS

WILLIAM PIVAR
College of the Desert

✸ SAUNDERS SURVIVAL SERIES

1979

W. B. SAUNDERS COMPANY · PHILADELPHIA · LONDON · TORONTO

W. B. Saunders Company: West Washington Square
Philadelphia, Pa. 19105

1 St. Anne's Road
Eastbourne, East Sussex BN21 3UN, England

1 Goldthorne Avenue
Toronto, Ontario M8Z 5T9, Canada

Survival Manual for Nursing Students   ISBN   0-7216-7252-3

Last digit is the print number: 9   8   7   6   5   4   3   2   1

Acknowledgments

I would like to thank the following people for their help in the preparation of this book: Mildred Nagler of the College of the Desert, Constance Bloom of Nicolet College, and Betty Grundy of Gogebic Community College, the three nurse educators who gave unselfishly of their time and effort in providing technical support; the staff of Howard Young Medical Center, Woodruff, Wisconsin, for their kind assistance; Douglas Garrison, Associate Professor of English at College of the Desert, whose proofreading and comments were invaluable; Luis Corona, Coordinator of Financial Aids at College of the Desert, for his assistance in the financial aid area; Amy Shapiro, the patient editor whose guidance helped me through the final days of writing; the many nurse educators who reviewed drafts and whose constructive criticism helped keep the book on the right track; and, lastly, Corinne Pivar, my wife and the photographer for this text, without whose constant aid this book would have never been written.

Contents

APPENDIX

Survival
Manual
for
Nursing
Students

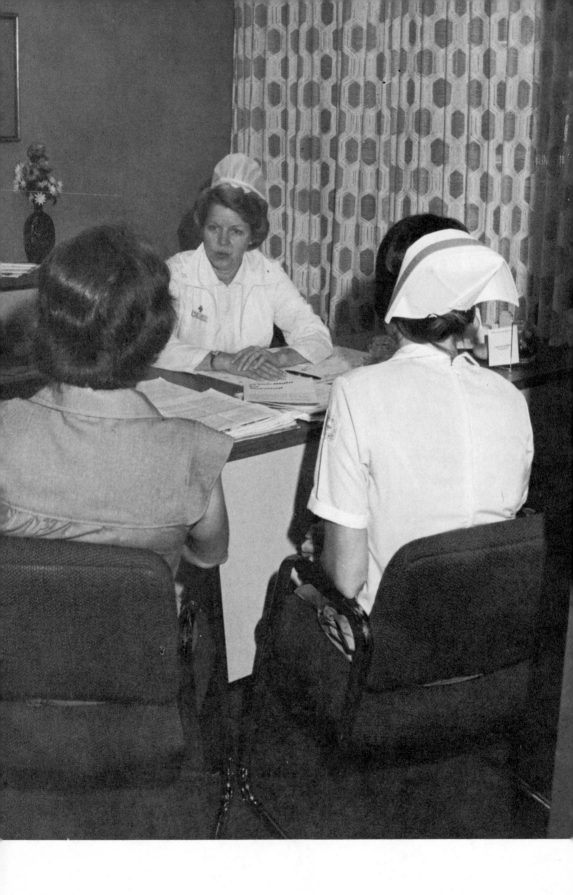

Chapter 1

Nursing and You

You're starting your nursing education. You probably have some mixed feelings and some apprehensions. You've looked forward to it for some time, but you're not sure what will be expected of you. You may even have some doubts about whether nursing is really for you.

WHAT IS NURSING?

Nursing is giving care. In order to be a nurse you must care. You must have a genuine concern for people if you wish to make nursing your life's work. Nursing also takes courage, emotional stability, and integrity.

In nursing you deal with all types of interesting people. Therefore, while nursing may be hard work it need never be boring if you care. Caring for others will help you to appreciate yourself as well as your patients. Nursing is a profession that encourages personal growth and awareness.

In nursing you must be flexible. You must adapt to new people and new situations. Patients don't adjust to nurses — nurses must adjust to patients.

Nursing involves more than just treatment. Prevention and rehabilitaiton are vital aspects of the nursing profession. It also involves much more than simply following orders from a doctor. In nursing you must be ready to accept and assume responsibility.

Graduation is not the end of your nursing education. Education in nursing is a lifelong process. There will be many opportunities to learn new skills. As a nurse you must adapt to the changing needs of society and the individual.

Some students regard nursing as "woman's work." But nursing is for people who are interested in science and who want to help and provide support for people. Some people think that men are more capable of scientific thought and that women are more "caring." This just is not so. Both men and women have the capacity to be professional and caring in their work.

THE NURSING TEAM

In your training you are going to learn to work as a member of a team. The team concept will be stressed throughout your training and your career. A head nurse or registered nurse (RN) acts as leader of the nursing team. The leader plans and guides the patient's care. He or she assigns tasks based on (1) the patient's needs and (2) the capabilities and personalities of the team members.

The nursing team consists of registered nurses, licensed practical nurses, vocational nurses (LPN–LVN), nursing aides, and orderlies. As a member of a nursing team you will be expected to contribute to discussions, question areas that are unclear, explain reasons for your own point of view, help other team members, and support decisions of the team when appropriate.

The nursing team is an integral part of an overall health team. The health team is responsible for the total care, treatment, and rehabilitation of the patient. In addition to the nursing team, the health team consists of physicians, therapists, psychologists or psychiatrists, dentists, and other supportive technicians and administrative workers as applicable. The health team has a singular goal, the total rehabilitation of the patient.

ROADS TO NURSING

There are three basic ways to prepare to become a registered nurse. Graduates from these programs all take the same state licensure examination to become a registered nurse.

Baccalaureate Degree. Bachelor's degree programs at colleges or universities usually last four years although some schools require five years. They grant a bachelor of science (BS) degree in nursing. This degree provides excellent preparation for graduate study and further specialization. (Some bachelor programs offer the opportunity for specialized training also.) Many administrative positions require a bachelor's degree, as do commissions in the armed forces.

Diploma Programs. These are usually three-year programs (although some take two years). They are given at a state approved school of nursing affiliated with an independent hospital. Emphasis is on the practical application of theory and direct patient care. Often the program is given in conjunction with a nearby college, where the required science courses are given.

Associate Degree. This degree is awarded for two years of study at a junior or community college. These are generally the shortest training programs available. Emphasis in these programs is on the technical aspects of patient care. General education as well as biological and behavioral science courses are required.

As a registered nurse you can be licensed in more than one state, either by examination or by endorsement of a license issued by another state board of nursing. There are a number of programs available for associate degree nurses and diploma nurses to enable them to earn a bachelor's degree. There is even an *external degree program,* for which normal class attendance is not required.

Advanced Degrees. To go on to graduate study you must have a bachelor's degree, and usually you are required to take the Aptitude Test of the Graduate Record Examination (GRE).

Master of Science in Nursing (MS). This program prepares leaders in specialized areas of nursing. The degree usually requires three to four semesters beyond the bachelor's degree for completion. Part-time students may spend three to five years earning their MS degree. A master's degree is frequently required for teaching, research positions, or independent practice.

Doctor of Nursing Science. Graduates assume complex leadership roles in the health care system and achieve a high level of competence in practice and research in a specialized area of nursing. The doctoral program usually takes two to three years of full-time effort beyond a master's degree.

LICENSED PRACTICAL NURSE

Licensed practical nurses (LPN, or, in Texas and California, licensed vocational nurse, LVN) perform duties that require nursing skills and techniques but not the education of an RN. They take blood pressure, temperature, and respiration rates. They administer medication, change dressings, and observe and report symptoms. They assist physicians and registered nurses in examining patients and carrying out nursing procedure. They may work in specialized areas such as intensive care, recovery rooms, and burn units. In most states a high school diploma is required for LPN preparation. The practical nursing programs can range from 9 to 18 months, but most usually last for one year.

The student must pass a state examination to be licensed as an LPN. Advancement is limited without continuing education. There are a number of programs that allow you to upgrade your LPN to RN status.

NURSE'S AIDE

Nurse's aides may receive on-the-job training and no formal schooling. However, a number of states now require a certificate from an approved nurse's aide course for employment. Nurse's aides work under the direction of an RN or LPN in providing direct patient care. They are involved in duties such as aiding in admission and discharge of patients, transporting of patients, taking of vital signs, feeding, patient skin care, making beds, etc.

PHYSICIAN'S ASSISTANT

These are new types of health care workers. A physician's assistant can take medical histories; write discharge summaries; perform detailed physical examinations; conduct visual, auditory, developmental, and laboratory tests; place casts on simple fractures; perform minor suturing and minor surgical procedures such as mole removal; and assist physicians in major surgery.

The physician's assistant program may require as little as two years of college for those with extensive medical backgrounds such as RNs and people with military service experience. Otherwise a four-year program is usually required.

In many states nurse practitioners, in addition to providing nursing care, assume a role similar to that of a physician's assistant. The length of training ranges from nine months to a year. Nurse practitioner training may be incorporated into a master's degree program. In this case training requires one to two years of study.

NURSE PRACTI- TIONER

Many completely different areas of activity are covered by the broad umbrella of nursing. For example, specialization may be according to age group of patients, such as neonatal, pediatric, adolescent, adult, and geriatric.

SPECIALTIES

The following is a partial list of subspecialties of nursing:

Ambulatory
Arthritis
Burn
Cancer (oncologic)
Cardiac–coronary care
Clinic nurse
Communicable disease
Community health nurse
Dermatologic
Diabetic
Emergency
Environmental
Family nurse practitioner
Family planning
Genetic counseling
Gynecologic
Home health nurse
In-service education nurse
Infection control
Intensive care
Maternity
Mental health
Metabolic
Neurosurgical
Nurse administrator
Nurse anesthetist
Nurse midwife
Nursery

Nursery–intensive care
Obstetric
Oncologic
Operating room
Orthopedic
Ostomy
Outpatient
Psychiatric
Public health nurse
Pulmonary
Recovery room
Rehabilitation
Respiratory
School nurse
Urologic dialysis

As your training progresses you will find out about these and other areas of specialization. Some specialization will be based on on-the-job experience; other fields require formal study.

JOB OPPOR- TUNITIES

While approximately 75 per cent of working nurses are employed in hospitals or long-term care facilities, you will find nurses in other job settings such as medical offices, schools, and research facilities.

Even industry employs *occupational health nurses* or *industrial nurses*. Besides providing emergency care, they are also concerned with prevention, recognition, and elimination of job-related accidents and illnesses. They counsel employees and recognize physical and emotional problems. They serve as the key health educator within a firm.

Private duty nurses give individualized care to patients. They are usually self-employed.

Community health nurses work in clinics, homes, or schools. They instruct patients and their families in health care and provide periodic treatment as prescribed by a physician.

GUIDING YOUR NURSING CAREER

As you can readily see, nursing offers a variety of opportunities to meet the needs of any person. You have individual needs different from those of others. Your nursing career can satisfy those needs. Just remember that you have the ability to guide your own career.

The first full-time nursing position a nurse takes often determines the direction of an entire working career, which may exceed 40 years. Students often spend less time in analyzing their career needs than they spend in deciding what kind of car to buy. When they buy a car they consider quality and priorities such as price, fuel economy, and so forth. After weighing these factors, they make an informed decision based on their own particular needs.

In the same manner as you buy a car you can plan your future. You can analyze your individual needs and choose the area of nursing that best satisfies those needs. It is possible to make an informed decision about the direction your career takes. You can control where you are going from here. Career choices are too important to leave to chance and also too important to be decided by parents, friends, or relatives. Your career direction should be your own.

Certainly there is more to life than just finishing your education and getting a job. Nevertheless, a great deal of your life is going to revolve around your career. If you can do a job well, you are going to be proud of the work you do, and you can expect to be happy in your work and in your life. That is what success is really all about.

Up to now you may have thought about nursing only in general terms. But as you can see, nursing encompasses a wide variety of specialties. As your education progresses and you have more nursing experience, you will see that certain areas stand out as being best suited to your individual needs. Use the following personal inventory to determine areas of interest that should be explored further.

1. What skills and special training do I now possess?

PERSONAL INVENTORY

With this question we reveal present skills, which might complement your educational training.

2. What do I consider to be my greatest assets?

3. A future employer would consider my greatest assets to be:

You should ask yourself, "How do these assets fit into my career plan?"

4. What are my weaknesses?

5. An employer would consider my greatest weakness to be:

There are two ways to deal with areas of weakness. One is to obtain additional training to strengthen yourself in these areas. The other is to choose a career that does not require proficiency in these areas.

6. What have I done in the past that I am really proud of?

7. Why?

8. What have I done that I would like to do again?

9. What work have I done in the past that I really enjoyed?

10. What specifically was there about this work that appealed to me?

11. What areas of my clinical experiences have I enjoyed the most?

12. Why?

13. What areas of my clinical experiences have I enjoyed the least?

14. Why?

15. What area of nursing study have I enjoyed the most?

16. Why?

17. What area of nursing study have I enjoyed the least?

18. Why?

The preceding questions are career area pointers. They relate to natural ability as well as to special interest.

19. Whom do I know who has the kind of nursing position I would like to have?

20. What specifically is there about these positions that I like?

21. Which nurse of my acquaintance do I admire most?

22. Why?

These questions are more specific career pointers. However, when you analyze what these jobs entail they may or may not be as attractive to you as they initially seemed.

23. What work have I done in the past that I have not liked . . . and why?

24. What nursing career areas am I definitely not interested in?

25. Why?

These questions point out "negative interests." Students often refuse to consider an area of specialization even if they dislike only one aspect of that specialty. Frequently they do not understand what the area actually entails. Talk with someone who works in a specialty that you think you don't like. You may be surprised to find the work more attractive than you had imagined.

26. What nursing skills or training do I wish I had?

27. Why?

These again are pointers to your own special interests.

28. How would I rate my verbal communication and listening ability?

29. How would I rate my written communication ability?

Possession of good skills in these areas is important in most administrative positions. Verbal skills are very important in people-oriented positions such as teaching.

30. Do I prefer to deal with people on a one to one basis or to work as a member of a group?

Certain specialties require individualized contact; other areas place great emphasis on group relations.

31. Do I enjoy travel?

32. Do I enjoy driving?

These questions will help you to determine whether you should make a nursing career choice that would require a great deal of travel, such as private duty nurse.

33. Would I prefer hospital work or outside work?

34. Would I prefer to have my day planned for me, or would I prefer to do my own planning and goal setting?

35. Would I prefer scheduled working hours?

36. Are the number of hours I work of major importance to me?

37. Do I want to be a member of a health team or carry my own patient load?

These questions reveal interests and attitudes that can significantly affect areas of specialization.

38. What, if any, are my physical limitations?

39. Do I like situations I am familiar with or would I prefer more challenge?

40. Would I prefer to know a great deal about a small area as a specialist or would I prefer a wider experience as a general duty nurse?

41. How important is job security to me?

If security is of prime consideration to you, you probably would not plan to be an independent private duty nurse. In your career choice you might want to trade off some degree of job satisfaction for greater security.

42. Am I ambitious?

If advancement is important to you, you will want to obtain additional educational experience so that you can progress to positions of greater responsibility. You should give consideration to postgraduate work if it is applicable.

43. Prior to answering these questions the area of nursing that most interested me was:

44. I am suited for this area because:

You are now in a much better position to analyze what may be the area of nursing that interests you most.

45. Other nursing areas that interest me are:

From the preceding questions you should have received some insight into other areas of interest.

46. What do I really want from my nursing career? (List in order of importance objectives such as job satisfaction, salary, working conditions, prestige, etc.).

By listing your priorities, you are in a good position to evaluate career areas suitable for you. Trade-offs often are necessary in making a choice, but by arranging your individual priorities you will be able to analyze how various career areas fit your individual needs and life style.

Perhaps the exercise of answering these questions simply reinforced your present plans. This would be a strong indication that you have chosen an area in which you are likely to be happy and successful.

If you are having difficulty in making decisions I suggest you go over your answers with a friend who is also in nursing training. A friend who listens to your answers can be as helpful as most career consultants, and you will save approximately $50 per hour.

You should consider taking the completed questions to one of your nursing instructors. Listen to his or her evaluation of your answers. But also remember that although others can help you in making a decision, the final choice is yours alone.

In your clinical work you will be exposed to many different areas of nursing. Find out as much as you can about each specialty so that you can make an informed decision about your career.

The National Student Nurses Association has many publications that can help you find the area of nursing that best fits your needs. Their booklet, "Thirteen Nurses — What They Say," can be particularly helpful. You can write for it to National Student Nurses Association, 10 Columbus Circle, Room 2330, New York, New York 10019.

Talk to nurses who are doing work that interests you. Generally people are flattered to be approached by someone who needs help in making important career decisions. You might find that a career area you considered glamorous loses some of its glitter, while other areas gain in excitement and challenge.

For information on any of the specialized areas of nursing, write National League for Nursing, 10 Columbus Circle, New York, New York 10019 and the American Nurses Association, 2420 Pershing Road, Kansas City, Missouri 64108.

You must be careful that your choice is not dictated by the fact that a particular career area requires little or no additional special training. If your career is not personally challenging, you could easily become a clock watcher whose high point of the day is the time he or she can go home.

SALARY

Don't make a choice based solely on financial reward. After a while you will find that money is less important than a job that remains challenging to you. Many nurses choose their first full-time job based on the amount of money offered. However, surveys of people who quit their first job show that money was listed as the main reason by fewer than 10 per cent. Reasons such as not being able to utilize specific knowledge were cited far more frequently. You can see from these data that while the recent graduate thinks that financial reward is extremely important, in fact it is not as significant as job satisfaction.

Most of us must spend a great deal of our lives working. If you don't like your work, you are going to be unhappy. When you hate the thought of getting out of bed and going to work, your career has become your prison. If this is the case, you can look forward to possible ulcers, hypertension, and even an early heart attack. Career happiness does affect your overall health. On the other hand, if you look forward to your work and enjoy it, you are going to be happy and are more likely to be healthy.

You are not going to find a career area in which every aspect brings great joy. Still, one can evaluate jobs in terms of a "happiness" quotient. I requested a large number of graduates to rate their job happiness on a scale of 1 to 10, and to supply me with income and other information. I discovered that there is no apparent correlation between income and happiness in terms of enjoying one's career. The old saying, "Money isn't everything," seems to hold true for job satisfaction. I also learned that among those graduates showing a high happiness quotient, the majority felt that their job fulfilled basic needs of recognition and self-esteem.

CHANGE AND FLEXIBILITY

We are in an age of swiftly changing technology. We can expect areas of nursing that are unknown today to be of major importance in the future. Additional training can open up whole new areas to you. You will also find that much of your training and experience in one specialty is applicable to other fields.

While you should start planning the direction you want your nursing career to take as soon as possible, you should realize that it is very possible your interests will change. Classes, instructors, friends, special interests, and experiences might cause you to modify or even completely reverse your original objectives. Your choices should not be inflexible. You should be open to change — but only when the change will better meet your own individual needs. You should not let anyone else dictate a career change.

In making your career and educational plans, you should consider all of the aspects covered, but most of all you should "consider."

NOTES

NOTES

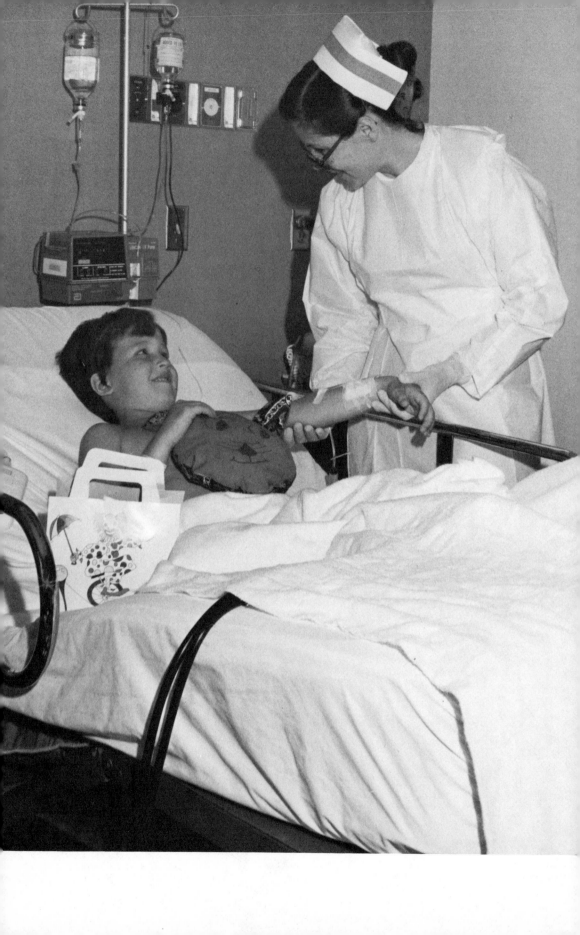

Chapter 2

Goal Setting

Today we hear a great deal about management by objective. This is nothing really new; it is simply goal setting. . .choosing realistic goals for the future and measuring our success in meeting them.

Without goals your life would have no real meaning. Many of us have known hard-working people who, shortly after retirement, seemed to wither and die in a very short time. These were people who worked a lifetime striving for goals. When they retired, they stopped reaching for greater improvement. They failed to set new goals for themselves, and without goals there is no purpose to life.

Goals are a blueprint, a map, a plan for your future. You wouldn't consider driving from Miami to Seattle without a road map. Why allow your life to drift without direction or purpose?

Without goals you are not going to really get started in any direction. Imagine yourself in a race without a finish line. You are not going to be motivated to keep on running without that line up ahead telling you how far you have to go to succeed. Meaningful goals are motivators that keep us striving for ever-greater achievements.

The nursing process as generally taught consists of four phases: assessment, planning, implementation, and evaluation. Goal setting is an integral part of each of these steps.

Assessment begins with a nursing history from which the nurse then determines patient needs. The nurse works with the patient to set goals for the patient. These can be

GOALS AND THE NURSING PROCESS

short range or long range objectives. The nurse and patient determine priorities and plan ways to reach these goals. The nursing plan is then implemented, and the results are evaluated.

This process of setting goals gives both the nurse and patient a sense of accomplishment. It is an individualized method of care, so the nurse and patient are assured that nursing does not become so routine that the unique talents of a nurse are wasted. By setting goals for patients and evaluating the results the nurse is really evaluating him or herself. Thus the nursing process strengthens nursing skills and results in improved patient care.

MOTIVATION   Just as goal setting can help patients, it can also help you. But it is not enough merely to set goals. You must choose objectives that you *want* to meet. The only real motivation for continued effort is self-motivation. You must strive because you want to achieve, not because someone else wants you to. Many people tend to adopt ideas of other people as their own. Since these ideas have no personal significance, such people are not strongly motivated to succeed. You must learn to "follow your own drummer."

The goals or objectives you set for yourself should be included in one of the following four categories:

New Learning Goals — A learning experience or accomplishment that is new to you.

Improvement Goals — An improvement in some project you are now doing, such as work habits or skills.

Problem Solving Goals — Obtaining a solution to a problem.

Personal Goals — Improving an area of human relations.

Goals don't have to be specifically related to a job. You might have goals for the school term such as:

a. I will complete the Health Care paper and turn it in at least one week prior to the May 1 deadline (new learning goal).
b. I will join at least one club or organization by the end of the term (personal goal).
c. I will attend at least five campus cultural events this term (concerts, art exhibits, and special lectures) (new learning goal).

   d. I will learn the names of at least eight fellow students in each of my classes and talk to them by name (personal goal).

   e. I will raise my grades in Anatomy from the current C to a B by the end of the term. I will accomplish this by readjusting my study schedule. (Problem solving goal and improvement goal).

   f. I will obtain no less than a 3.6 grade point average this term (improvement goal).

   g. I will make a positive contribution to every post-clinical conference (personal goal).

Your plans should always be stated in specific, measurable terms. It must be absolutely clear whether a goal has or has not been met.

Make a list of your goals and identify them as personal, problem solving, improvement, or new learning. By writing them down you are consciously defining them. This exercise triggers self-motivation and makes it more difficult to concoct excuses about why your goals were not met.

You already have a specific career goal: You want to be a nurse. As you know, within the broad heading of nursing are many specialties requiring additional training and/or experience. There is also a broad spectrum of career choices within each specialty.

Nursing can be a first step toward other careers such as hospital administration, physical or occupational therapy, and pharmacy. Within the health field are many careers that would benefit by your nursing training. Even if you decide to leave nursing for another health related career, your nursing training has not been wasted. It will serve as a solid base to make you better at whatever health area you enter.

ONE STEP AT A TIME— YOUR INTERIM GOALS

You may have a particular specialty in mind at this time. You may even have alternative areas of interest. Use your specific career goal to help you define the steps, or interim goals, that you must take along the way. These steps should follow a logical sequence. They may be appropriate to several career areas. For example, becoming an RN is the starting point for most medical-surgical specialties. A master's degree in nursing science could prepare you for a number of careers in research, administration, nursing education, or any one of many specialties.

If you are undecided about the area of nursing you want to pursue, whenever possible your interim goals should be applicable to several career choices. But be sure that your steps lead you to a specific destination; otherwise you may attain many short-term goals but fail to achieve your ultimate objective.

So you see how important it is to map out your path. What goals should be attained to meet your career goal, and in what order should they be reached?

In making any career plan you should analyze what you will actually be *doing* when you reach your goal. Forget about titles — they don't describe the actual job. Talk to people who hold these titles to find out what the job entails. Armed with this information, you'll be able to determine what preparation — training, schooling, etc. — you need for the career you're interested in.

Answer the following questions to help you in your career plan.

FORMAL EDUCATIONAL GOALS
1. What education (degrees and/or special courses) do I need to attain my career goal?

WORKING SKILL GOALS
2. What skill improvement is necessary for me to reach my career goal?

3. What additional skills can I learn that will help me to reach my career goal?

EXPERIENCE GOALS
4. What additional experience will help prepare me for my career goal? (Be specific.)

The needs that these questions reveal are really steps or plateaus to reach in your career ascent. You have decided where you want to be in 20 years; now you are simply deciding the best way of getting there.

Many different types of training can be utilized for the same career. For example, if you want to become a nurse educator, your training might be in such widely diverse areas as geriatrics, nurse anesthetist, nurse practitioner, etc.

Let's say that you've decided that you want to be a nurse educator specializing in geriatrics. You are now enrolled in an associate degree nursing program. Your path might be as follows:

14 yrs.	I will obtain a full-time staff position in a school of nursing.
12 yrs.	I will obtain a part-time teaching position in the geriatric care area at a school of nursing.
11 yrs.	I will obtain a Master of Science degree in nursing with specialization in geriatric care by continuing my part-time education.
6 yrs.	I will obtain my bachelor's degree in nursing science by continuing my education on a part-time basis.
2 yrs.	I will obtain full-time employment in a geriatric care facility as an RN.
2 yrs.	I will obtain my associate degree in nursing.
1 month	I will obtain part-time and vacation employment in an institution specializing in geriatric care.

The full-time teaching position in geriatrics is your career goal; the others are interim goals, or steps. Each of these intermediate achievements can be further broken down to many lesser goals. As an example, the final step (to obtain full-time employment as a nurse educator) might consist of the following tasks:

    a. I will develop a résumé and cover letter for a position as teacher of geriatric nursing.
    b. I will obtain lists of nursing schools and mail out at least 200 résumés.
    c. I will personally visit at least 5 of these schools.
    d. I will telephone at least 30 of these schools.
    e. I will attend at least 3 professional nurse educator meetings and/or conventions.

Goals should be re-evaluated periodically since the relevance of a goal may change. Don't make a goal a "commandment." Be flexible as you and your needs change. Set realistic timetables for accomplishing your goals, and review and re-evaluate them along with your plans.

MAKING TIME WORK FOR YOU

A key to success in meeting goals is the management of time.

A dozen people with the same amount of time to utilize may have widely varying levels of accomplishment within that time. Ben Franklin learned to account for his time through a series of daily goals. Each night he would make a list of his aims for the next day. One item might simply be to devote a period of time to some endeavor. He then reviewed his accomplishments for the day that had just passed and compared them with the goals he had set the night before. If he had not met a goal he asked himself why. By writing his goals he was able to evaluate his daily accomplishments critically. He didn't like being critical about his own abilities, since his pride sometimes suffered in the process, but by using his list as a motivator, he maximized his time — as evidenced by his success as printer, inventor, writer, publisher, and statesman.

You may not be another Ben Franklin, but if you set daily goals and follow them, you will find you are able to get a great deal more accomplished in one day than you felt possible. An old Chinese proverb states: "A journey of a thousand miles starts with the first step." By setting daily goals you will reach your intermediate goals, and if these are relevant to your career goal, then that too is within your reach.

Goals may be redefined, and routes to them may change, but without goals, you will drift aimlessly. Don't leave to chance that which is within your grasp.

NOTES

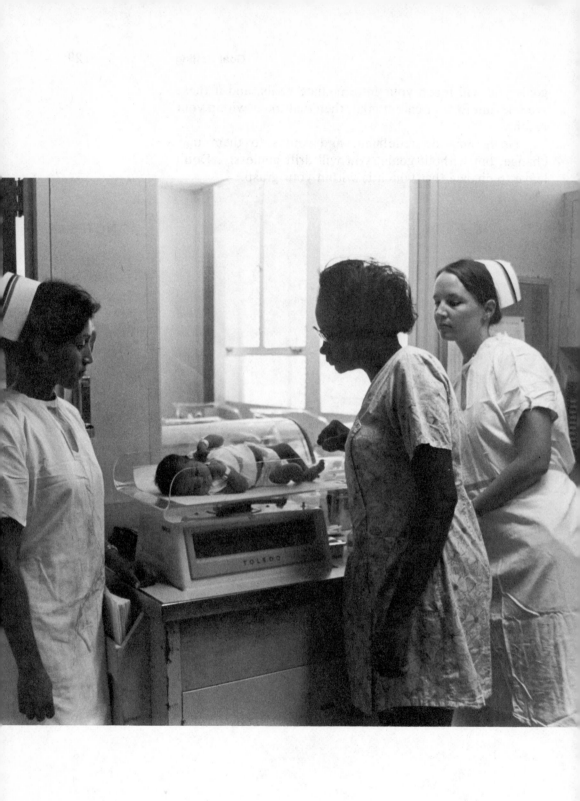

Chapter 3

Preparing for Success

Success requires motivation. It is not enough to wish for something; you must be motivated to work for it.

If your goals are meaningful to you, they will serve as motivators. If, however, your goals mean little to you, it is going to be hard to get enthusiastic about your nursing education. If this is the case, a re-evaluation of goals is in order.

We tend to identify with our dominant peer group and to pattern ourselves after our friends. If you associate with people who are motivated to achieve their goals, you will find that they reinforce your own enthusiasm. If your friends are apathetic and have a "what's the use, the whole world is going to hell" attitude, you can expect this negativism to affect you. You can see the importance of choosing friends and groups that can share your desire to achieve and inspire you to grow.

A positive attitude is necessary for motivation and success. If you doubt your own abilities, your level of effort will reflect this lack of confidence. Unfortunately, most of us tend to be more negatively motivated than we are positively motivated. Dr. Maxwell Maltz points this out in his excellent book *Psycho-Cybernetics*.

How many times have you heard students say, "I'm lousy at math." By repeating it often enough, they come to believe it. No matter how much instruction they receive, they are unable to learn because they have become negatively reinforced. By saying you can't do something and then failing when you try, you create a self-fulfilling prophecy.

You can overcome your tendency to be negatively motivated. When my son first tried water skis he fell flat on his face. When he got back to the dock he said, "Did you see me? I almost got up on my skis!" He was positively motivated by an attempt that most people would have viewed as a disaster. He wanted to succeed and saw some positive results in his first attempt. Because he continued to believe that he could do it, he was inspired to keep trying until he was successful.

ROLE PLAYING

Role playing can be used to cultivate a positive frame of mind. Actors sometimes find that when they are playing a role it affects their personal life. They have become the character they are playing. In these cases the effects of role playing are unconscious. It is possible to consciously work at becoming the person you would like to be by "acting the part."

PREPARING FOR SUCCESS

As an aid to role playing, list the characteristics you would like to have:

1. _____

2. _____

3. _____

4. _____

5. _____

6. _____

For each of these traits, list at least two situations in which you feel you have exhibited these characteristics:

1. a. _____

   b. _____

2. a. _____

   b. _____

3. a. _____

   b. _____

4. a. _____

   b. _____

5. a. _____

   b. _____

6. a. _____

   b. _____

Now you can see that the role you wish to play isn't really so different from who you are now. Make a conscious effort to do things the way this person you wish to be would do them. In your daily life ask yourself how the character you are playing (which after all is nothing but an unexpressed facet of your personality) would handle the situation. After a while you will find you are no longer acting. You have discovered that the character you were playing was really you all along.

In the song "Whistle a Happy Tune" from the musical *The King and I,* Anna sings, "When I fool the people I fear, I fool myself as well." What Anna is saying, of course, is that by role playing, she convinces herself as well as others that she is unafraid.

People who think that they cannot dance well have been known to do so while under hypnosis. Hypnosis purges the mind of past failures that serve as negative reinforcers. If you can think of yourself as a success, if your self-image is positive, then you're well on the road to reaching your objectives.

A new face can change a person's self-image. Many people have resorted to cosmetic surgery as the only way to bolster their regard for themselves. After surgery their self-image changed along with their exterior appearance. They liked themselves. With this change they found whole new avenues open to them.

Plastic surgery does nothing more than change one's "packaging" a little.

Certainly nothing so drastic is necessary to help you to feel more positively about yourself. Like growth, self-esteem is a continuing process. In your nursing career you will have many opportunities to learn to value yourself, your work, and other people. Be open to these lessons. As your opinion of your own worth changes and as you learn to respect yourself, you'll find that others will respect you, too.

POSITIVE REINFORCE-MENT

Another technique for increasing self-esteem is to talk about your successes, no matter how small. Tell a friend, your spouse, your parents — someone who will be supportive of you. The pleasure of sharing your triumphs with someone close to you will provide positive reinforcement that not only will help your self-image but also will provide incentive for future successes. You will find yourself on a highly productive cycle: the more you achieve, the better your self-image will be; and the better your self-image, the more you'll be able to achieve. As your grades improve, you will strive for even better grades. Nothing seems to help success like success.

As an aid to a good self-image, list what you believe to be your strong personal assets and your reasons for considering them so:

1. _____

_____

Reasons: _____

_____

2. _____

_____

Reasons: _____

_____

3. _____

_____

Reasons: _____

_____

It is not egotistical to like yourself. The fact that you have faults shouldn't stop you from liking yourself. We all have imperfections, but this doesn't mean we're not worth-while human beings.

Liking yourself does not mean that you should ignore your faults. Only by recognizing them and admitting that these are problem areas can you work to improve your character.

The simple act of listing what you consider to be your faults or problem areas and then listing ways of improving will serve as a starting point for change and will bring your faults into proper perspective.

Personal problems are:

1. _____

_____

Ways to improve: _____

_____

_____

_____

2. _____

_____

Ways to improve: _____

_____

_____

_____

3. _____

_____

Ways to improve: _____

_____

_____

_____

No one likes to be criticized. We must learn to take criticism in a positive manner. Unfortunately, some faculty members may point out your shortcomings in a negative rather than a positive way. Don't take this personally. Even if you feel that criticism is unjustified, treat it as a guide for further improvement. Don't let anyone make you feel inadequate as a person. You don't know everything yet, but the skills and lessons that you learn at school will extend your abilities in many areas that you now find difficult.

If you were not a person of ability you would not have gone as far as you have. The fact that you have been admitted into a highly competitive nursing program shows that others regard you as a person of great worth. The attitude that you can succeed and, more important, that you *will* succeed means far more than heredity, environment, or even I.Q. You are capable of succeeding in both nursing and life.

NOTES

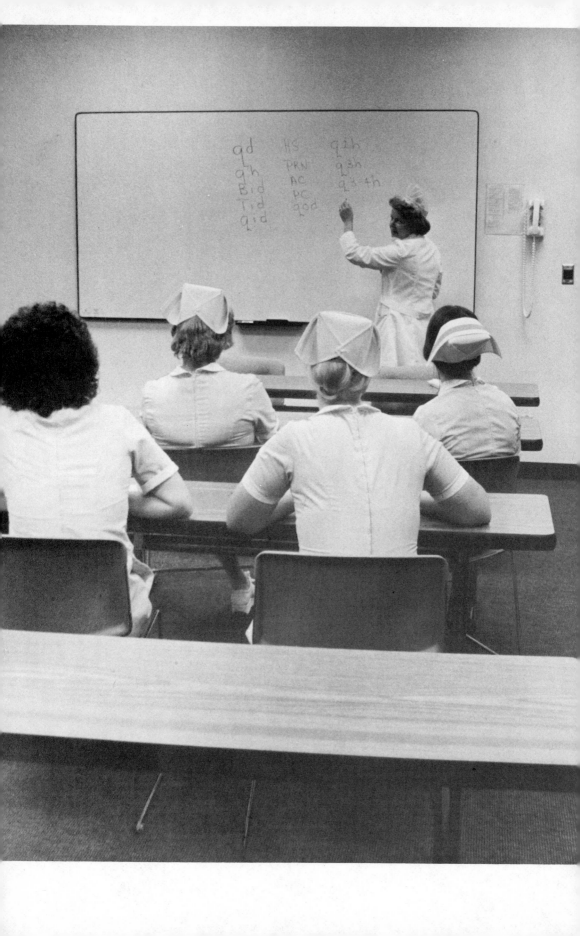

Chapter 4

Planning Your Curriculum

Your nurse training will probably take place five days per week. You will probably spend from 6 to 15 hours per week in classes and from 6 to 24 hours per week in clinical experience at a hospital. These hours vary based on individual school, type of program, and semester of training.

Regardless of what program you are enrolled in, you can expect classes in the following areas:

Anatomy.   The study of human organs and organ systems. In many anatomy courses, students dissect a mammal that is comparable in structure to humans.

Microbiology.   (High school or college chemistry is usually a pre-requisite.) This course stresses diseases produced by microorganisms. It includes an introduction to microorganism classification, cytology (biology of the formation, structure, and function of cells), physiology (science of life processes), growth, reproduction, sterilization, disinfection, and the applied fields of microbiology. Bacteriological techniques are emphasized in the laboratory.

Physiology.   General principles of life processes with emphasis on the healthy human body.

Some schools require courses in the following areas:

Child Growth and Development.   Study of physical, social, and emotional development from infancy through adolescence.

SUBJECTS OF STUDY

39

Psychology. Study of human behavior, including motivation, emotions, and adjustment as well as abnormal behavior patterns.

Sociology. The study of social problems and how they affect human relationships.

NURSING COURSES

Your nursing courses will provide direct clinical experience in a health care setting as well as classroom education. Theoretical and laboratory aspects of nursing usually are taught concurrently. Titles of nursing courses vary, but the substance is as follows:

Fundamentals of Nursing. This introductory course includes the professional, legal and moral responsibilities of nursing. You will learn the basics of the nursing process, which you will utilize throughout your career. In your clinical training, you will learn assessment (identifying and determining needs of the patient), planning (setting goals), implementation of plans, and evaluation of results.

Mental health concepts, in the context of basic human needs and communication techniques, will be introduced.

Your experiences with patients provide an opportunity to develop skill and confidence in the application of concepts and principles learned in the classroom.

Medical-Surgical Nursing. This course is taught at the introductory as well as the advanced level. Topics include phases of illnesses, pharmacology, diet, and rehabilitation. You will learn the relationship of the various components of the nursing process. Your clinical experience will help you to develop patient care skills and confidence in your abilities.

Acute Care Nursing. This course emphasizes the application of the nursing process to patients with acute, traumatic, or critical illnesses. Laboratory experiences will include work in emergency room and intensive care units.

In addition, the following nursing courses may be offered at your school:

Psychiatric Nursing. Emphasizes mental health concepts and principles as they apply to patients in hospitals, home, and community.

Maternity Nursing. Biologic and social science principles applied to the care of maternity patients and their families. Emphasis placed on the role of the nurse in the maintenance of family health and the prevention of disease.

Pediatric Nursing. Study of infancy, childhood and adolescence. Pharmacology and nutrition and concepts of growth and development are integrated throughout the course. Emphasis is placed on the role of the nurse in promoting and maintaining child health and effective parenting.

Knowledge of the following terms will be helpful, particularly if you are enrolled in a baccalaureate degree program.

Lower Division Courses. General introductory studies, of a preparatory and survey nature, normally taken during the first two years of college.

General Education Courses (or Breadth Courses). Lower division courses that are required for graduation. These subjects (e.g., English, Speech, Sociology, Psychology, Ethics, Anthropology, etc.) will help you to understand and appreciate the arts and sciences as well as provide experience in the ability to analyze, make decisions, and communicate. These courses are people-oriented rather than directly related to a vocation. They help to make you a well-rounded person.

Upper Division Courses. In-depth courses normally taken during the junior and senior years.

Electives. Non-required courses for a major or degree. They are used to fill in the total number of credits required for graduation.

Major. Primary field of study or specialization. A major consists of a specified number of upper division subjects in a particular area of study. Units used for a major generally cannot be used to meet general education requirements.

Minor. A secondary field of study, consisting of a lesser number of credits in a field of study.

Associate Degree (AN). A two-year degree, normally obtained from a junior college. Approximately 60 semester units or 90 quarter units are required (includes general education requirements).

Bachelor's Degree (BSN). The traditional four-year degree, requiring approximately 120 semester units or 180 quarter units.

$$\text{Quarter Unit} \times \tfrac{2}{3} = \text{Semester Unit}$$
$$\text{Semester Unit} \times 1\tfrac{1}{2} = \text{Quarter Unit}$$

TYPES OF COURSES AND DEGREES

Master's Degree (MSN). Varies from about 50 to 60 semester units or 75 to 90 quarter units (based on school and area of study). Requires approximately two years of study beyond a bachelor's degree. A thesis or special project is normally required.

Doctoral Degree (PhD). Normally takes two to three years beyond the master's degree. Generally requires courses plus a thesis.

CREDIT REQUIREMENTS
With approximately 120 semester units to be earned for a bachelor's degree (or approximately 60 for an associate degree) you must carry an average of 15 units per semester. Your school catalog will explain your exact credit requirements.

You should also check your school catalog for general educational requirements. Assume your school requires 40 units of general education courses. Since these are considered lower division courses and are therefore taken during the first two years, you will have approximately 20 semester units of electives for these two years. You should try to get your general education courses out of the way as soon as possible.

ELECTIVES
In diploma and associate degree nursing programs, few electives are offered. You are being prepared for a staff position as a registered nurse. Future specialization will be based on additional training or experience. Electives *are* part of the baccalaureate program, so some specialization is possible.

Within your general education courses you will have some freedom to choose. For example, your school might require four courses in the social science area. Your choices might be history, political science, philosophy, psychology, and sociology. For nursing you might consider one course in sociology and three in psychology. While this is more psychology than will be required for your nursing degree, it will nevertheless help you in your career. A course in political science might be very interesting, but it will do little to make you a better nurse. When you have choices you should analyze them in terms of which one will be of greatest value in your nursing career. If in doubt, talk to one of your nursing instructors.

You may have taken a course at another institution that has the same or similar title as one that is required in nursing school. It's important to realize that there is no uniformity among schools as to course titles or content. Two entirely different courses could have the same title, and two similar courses could have widely differing titles. If your present school does not consider a course you took elsewhere to be equivalent to their required course, they are unlikely to give credit for it.

Don't waste your electives. Use them to reinforce your career goal. You may be very interested in basketweaving, but is it really going to help your career? Wouldn't an additional science course or some sociology, psychology, and anthropology courses be much more relevant to your plans?

PLANNING YOUR CURRICULUM

In planning your schedule don't try to bunch up all your classes one right after the other in three days in order to have two days off. Leave some breathing space. Allow for some time to relax, study, organize, and eat. Some students take classes they are not particularly interested in because these courses fit into this type of compact schedule that gives them long weekends.

After you've made some friends on campus, you'll get a lot of advice such as, "Take a course from Smith because he gives no assignments and everyone gets at least a B"; or "Don't take classes from Jones unless you don't mind working your head off for a C." Everyone is going to have opinions about instructors, and you will hear many different views of the same instructor. Most instructors have some students who feel they are the greatest and some who feel they are the worst. Don't accept other people's opinions. You're going to school to learn to think for yourself; try to be your own person now.

In the same vein, don't take classes just because they're easy. An easy course or teacher does little to improve you. Time and money are being invested in your education; make the most of this investment.

If you hope to attend graduate school or specialist training programs, find out the *GPA* (grade point average) that is required for admittance. This will give you a goal to aim for, which is an incentive for better work.

Even if you're not interested in graduate school, you must maintain a certain GPA to stay in school and to graduate. Generally, 2.0 is the minimum GPA.

Some courses are graded on a *pass-fail* basis. These are not computed into your grade point average. If your grade point average needs bolstering, such a course will not help you.

In Chapter 2 we discussed the importance of choosing your own goals, making your own career decisions. But sometimes students mistakenly reject all suggestions from others, even when these ideas reflect the student's own interests. Perhaps your parents have encouraged you to study nursing. You may feel that this decision has been forced upon you. Certainly this may be the case, and if you find that nursing is not for you, then by all means change your course of study. But are you sure that you're not interested in nursing — or are you merely trying to assert your independence or to show defiance? Don't throw away this great opportunity until you've taken time to examine your motives fully.

It is possible to be enrolled at more than one college at the same time. *Dual enrollment* normally does not require any special permission. Its purpose is to pick up a required course that cannot otherwise be taken because of a conflict in schedules. You should, however, check with your registrar first. If a course at another school does not duplicate in content the required course at your school, you might not receive credit for it.

It may not be necessary to actually take the full number of credits required for graduation. You can take the *CLEP test* (College Level Examination Program) to receive up to two years' college credit for what you already know. These tests are given at many colleges and universities. The CLEP program itself does not grant credit, so check with your registrar to be sure that CLEP scores are accepted at your school.

Many schools give college credits for military service. In addition, courses you may have taken in the service may be worth college credit. The *Guide to the Evaluation of Educational Experiences in the Armed Forces,* published by the American Council on Education, lists the recommended college credits for various government schools and correspondence courses. Many schools follow this guide.

If you feel that you know the subject matter of a course, many schools allow you to challenge the course by examination. This means that with permission you can take an examination to receive credit for a course without actually taking the course. Information about challenging a course is available from your school registrar and your school nursing department.

Your curriculum decisions must be made by you. No one else should make them for you. Make your decisions based on your own needs, and you will find your course work to be a satisfying and enriching experience.

NOTES

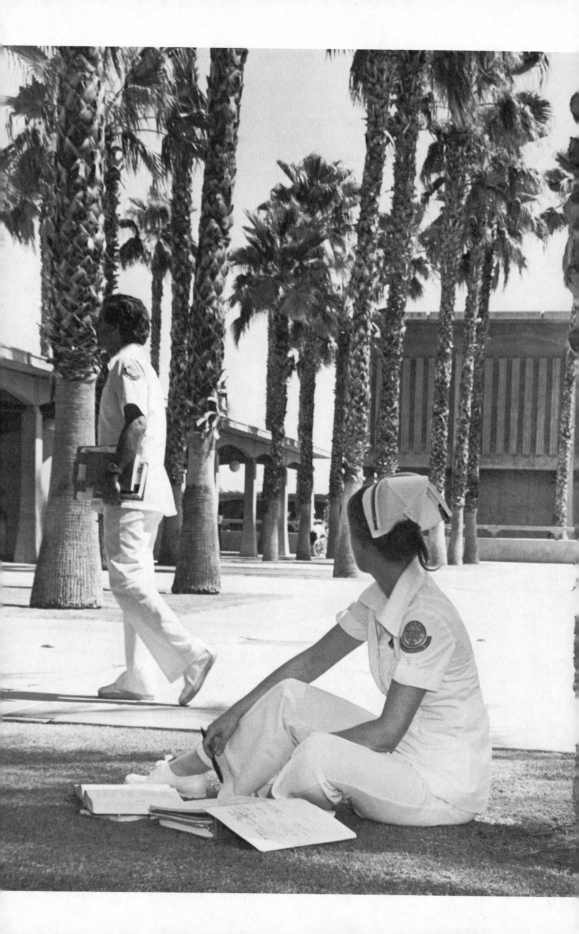

Chapter 5

How to Study

It's easy to get through high school without developing good study techniques. Many of your classmates in high school had no intention of going on for further education, and many of them were not motivated. In this type of environment, a moderate amount of study is sufficient to get you into a college or a nursing program. Now, however, you are going to have to prove yourself against far greater academic competition.

You are entering an exacting course of study. What you learn in nursing school will determine your competence for the rest of your working career. What you fail to learn properly can create problems throughout your working life.

Admittance to graduate schools and specialist training programs is limited. Even if you are not interested in further study at present, goals do change. A good grade point average will keep additional options open to you.

You might also find that studying on a "get by" basis may not be enough when you come to your important state board examination.

In this chapter you will learn how to make the most of the time available for study. Your first task is to set up a study schedule; your second is to learn the fine art of studying.

How should you allocate your study time? Make a chart covering a full week, as shown in the accompanying diagram. Fill in the chart with your class and lab time. If you are working, your work hours should also be shown. The areas that are blank can be devoted either to study or to other activities.

It's important to designate specific days and times for the study of each subject. The more precise your schedule is, the more likely you are to stick to it. A loosely organized study plan is easier to break than a carefully constructed one. A general rule of thumb is to set aside at least two study hours for each hour of academic class time. If you're taking 15 hours of classes, you should plan to study for 30 hours. This means that you must devote 45 hours per week to your education.

Not all courses require two hours of study for every hour in class; but some may require a great deal more. As the school term progresses, you will find that adjustments will be necessary. The amount of study time for each course might change, but be very careful about reducing the total time allocated for study.

Study should be your number one priority. If it becomes necessary to change your study schedule, you must be sure you are able to gain back any study time by taking the time from some other activity.

Daily Class and Study Schedule

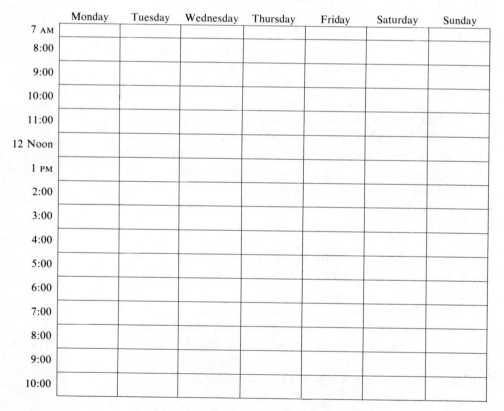

	Monday	Tuesday	Wednesday	Thursday	Friday	Saturday	Sunday
7 AM							
8:00							
9:00							
10:00							
11:00							
12 Noon							
1 PM							
2:00							
3:00							
4:00							
5:00							
6:00							
7:00							
8:00							
9:00							
10:00							

Your schedule should make every hour important. In addition to time set aside for study, budget time for eating and sleeping and for recreation and relaxation activities. Recreation is a necessary part of your total system, and you should plan for it just as you plan for study. By sticking to your study plan, you will enjoy your relaxation time much more because you won't feel guilty. You will know that you have earned the time off.

Periods between classes and short breaks can be very valuable. Schedule that time just as you do the larger time periods. Some people find that the best time to review their notes is right after class. Others like to study their notes from the previous day just before a class, so that they are prepared for any class discussions. You may want to use these short breaks for relaxation, to stretch or take a walk or have a cup of coffee. Experiment a bit until you find a schedule that suits you. You'll soon discover your own natural rhythm of working and relaxing.

Working full-time while you're attending nursing school is a very demanding proposition. Your study time will have to be adjusted around your work schedule as well as your class schedule. Because this reduces the net time available for study, you may find you have to use every available minute, including lunch and coffee breaks at work. A great deal of careful planning is necessary, but many people find that studying during these short periods quickly becomes a habit.

Even the time spent in commuting from work, school, or hospital can be utilized. When you are driving you can use the time to try to recall and reconstruct the last lecture or laboratory session (always, of course, giving the major part of your concentration to the road). This exercise in recall will reinforce your learning. Driving to work can also be a good time to listen to tapes of lectures.

Married students should not neglect their families. While education is important, it should not be at the expense of normal family life. Just as you incorporate relaxation into your schedule, you should set aside time for family activities. If you feel your education is seriously affecting your family life, you should consider revising your schedule. After all, your family life can seriously affect your education. Difficulties at home can make it hard to concentrate, and your work may suffer. Happiness at home can help you to maintain the energetic and positive frame of mind needed for a good education.

Naturally the best time to study is while you are alert. Don't plan on using late hours when you have to force yourself to stay awake. A well-thought out schedule can eliminate those 2:00 AM cram sessions.

Later in this chapter we will discuss the value of spreading out your studying time (see page 54). Your schedule should provide for study periods of no more than an hour at a time for a given subject. Thirty to 45 minutes has been found to be the ideal study time for most people.

Whenever possible you should avoid studying closely related subjects in sequence, as this can lead to confusion. For example, schedule your sociology study period to follow your chemistry study. This alternation between "hard" and "soft" sciences will refresh you and help you to retain what you learn.

Make a list of your courses and rate them according to difficulty. Arrange your study periods so that your work on the less demanding subjects is interspersed between study of the harder subjects.

You may want to schedule your toughest assignment first so that you'll get a feeling of accomplishment when you're done. Many students find that this method makes the rest of their work seem much easier.

In addition to planning for your daily and weekly assignments, term projects such as papers or additional books to be read should be worked into your study plan. By allotting a certain amount of time each day for long-term work, you'll avoid the all too common pitfall of trying to write a 20-page paper or prepare a complex project in one night at the end of the semester, when you should really be reviewing for final exams.

A carefully planned schedule prevents things from piling up, and when work piles up, a pressure situation is created. Generally, studying under pressure is not very effective. When you are not under pressure, the work becomes more interesting; and when there is interest, retention is increased.

A study plan should be detailed. It should cover not only what subject is to be studied but also the area of the subject and how it is to be studied. Therefore, in addition to the general weekly plan for the term you should have a refined plan for specific days. For many of us, an undetailed study plan represents a great temptation to spend too much time on areas of interest within a general subject and to avoid completely other aspects of the course. Since you usually do better in the subjects you're interested in, these are probably the areas that need the *least* amount of your study time. For example, if you're especially fascinated by circulatory physiology, you probably understand it better than some facet of the subject that you find less intriguing, such as renal physiology. What this means is that you probably need to spend more time on renal physiology. If your schedule reads simply "Study physiology," which area would you be likely to turn to?

A detailed plan for one day's study might look like the one shown in the box. By adhering to your schedule you will find yourself unable to avoid unpleasant tasks. Procrastination will become exceedingly difficult. And who knows — you may even learn to enjoy topics that you thought were too difficult for you or too dull. Just as you tend to do well in subjects that interest you, you'll find that your interest in a subject increases as your understand it better. Your hard work will be reflected in your satisfying sense of accomplishment as well as in your grades.

Tuesday, February 27

8:00–12:00 Noon — Clinical
12:00–12:45 PM — Lunch
12:45–1:00 PM — Review Microbiology prior to class.
1:55–2:00 PM — Review Anatomy prior to class.
3:00–4:00 PM — Review lecture notes Chapter 1–4. Microbiology (1/2 hour). Scan and read Chapter 5 (1/2 hour).
4:00–5:00 PM — Anatomy: study section 4 for quiz.
5:00–5:30 PM — Review clinical lab manual part 4.
5:30–6:30 PM — Dinner
6:30–7:30 PM — Prepare draft of case study assignment for Nursing 101.
7:30–8:30 PM — Meet with Sally and Ed to go over clinical experience in preparation for tomorrow's pre-conference.
8:30–10:00 PM — R/R (Rest and Relaxation)

Your schedule should not be so inflexible that it cannot be changed. In fact, periodically you should re-evaluate your weekly study plan. Ask yourself whether you're giving enough time to subjects. Is your study time effective? What can be done to improve your study techniques? While a study plan must allow some flexibility, you must remember that if you allow it to be changed too readily, it will soon be forgotten.

Without a study plan, you'll probably fall behind on your assignments. When you fall behind, the only solution is to cram. Even if you manage to pass the course this way, information learned quickly is also forgotten quickly. This can lead to major problems if this information is needed as the basis for further study or is directly relevant to nursing care. Remember that you're in school to learn, not merely to pass exams.

If you have personal problems, try to put them out of your mind while you're studying. A minute or two spent thinking of something very pleasant will help greatly in reducing anxiety prior to studying. Some students find that a few minutes of physical exercise prior to studying helps them to put their personal problem on the "back burner" so that effective study is possible. If you find that personal problems or worries are making it impossible for you to concentrate on your work, seek help from a sympathetic counselor. Talk to your minister or pastor, the school psychologist, or even a mature and understanding friend. We'll discuss adjustment problems further in Chapter 9.

PHYSICAL SETTING

Choose your place of study with care. One place is not just as good as another. You should have a comfortable, well-lighted area for study, with as few distractions as possible.

Your place of study should allow you to write easily, so that you can take notes and spread out papers and books. (This generally precludes studying in bed or on an easy chair.)

Avoid using a desk light with only one fluorescent bulb. The flicker can cause eye fatigue. Normally two-bulb fluorescents are adjusted to eliminate flicker.

While dormitories offer many social advantages that are important in your development as a well-rounded person, they are generally very poor places to study. The more distractions an area offers, the more difficult it is to study.

Your study room should not be a place where friends can reach you readily, either in person or by phone. It should not be in proximity to a TV, since an interesting program can easily lead you to stray from your study plan. Distractions and interruptions lessen the effectiveness of the time you spend in study.

On a nice day, the temptation to study outdoors can be almost irresistible. But you'll find that the great outdoors offers too many distractions. Birds singing, bugs crawling by, people strolling across a field, airplanes flying over-head — all these interesting events conspire to draw your attention from your work. Even a light breeze can set all your papers in motion, and the glare from the sun can make reading difficult. I'm sure you can think of many other disadvantages to studying outdoors; in fact, everything that makes being outside enjoyable and attractive also makes it the wrong place for you to concentrate on your work.

Avoid study spots that are too warm, as high temperatures can make you very sleepy. Your study location should be comfortable but not so comfortable as to induce sleep. You'll find that a heavy meal before studying will also tend to put you to sleep. When you find yourself getting tired, take a quick break. Even a slight change of activity such as a short walk or a shower will frequently revive you.

STUDY AIDS

The tools you will generally need for study are a regular dictionary, medical dictionary, textbook, colored pens, and a notebook. Scissors, cellophane tape, and a ruler are also useful. Cultivate the habit of studying with a pen or pencil in your hand so that you'll be more likely to underline important passages and take notes.

Have you ever noticed that when someone sits down at a table in a crowded library, about half the people at the table look up? People who are trying to study welcome an opportunity to be distracted. Those who do not look up are those who do not let outside events affect their train of thought. You must learn to ignore external stimuli while you're concentrating.

One hour of study is not necessarily as valuable as another. If you were to study a subject for 10 hours straight you would get far more out of the first hour than from the tenth hour. After a while you would have trouble keeping your mind on the work. You would find yourself using up the time without really studying. It has been found that it is easier to concentrate for shorter periods of time. Therefore, your retention is much better when you "spread out" the learning process. Study a subject for ½ hour a day for seven days, and your retention of the material will be much greater than if you spend 3½ hours studying at one stretch. In addition, the material that you work through gradually, in ½ hour stages, will stay with you longer than the information you race through on the night before the exam.

You can effectively break up your study time by taking a short rest every 30 to 45 minutes. Get a drink of water, write a short letter, or do any minor personal chore. After the break, start work on a new subject. This technique serves to revitalize your interest.

The effectiveness of study is directly related to your interest in what you are studying. Have you ever found yourself reading a text and suddenly realizing that you have no idea what you've been reading? Have you ever lost your place only to find that you don't know what you have read and what you haven't? Your mind wandered off while you continued to read on, line by line, without absorbing anything.

When you read a novel, your mind seldom wanders. You're interested and pay attention. When you're finished, you can describe what you've read in great detail. Often you vividly remember what you have read for years afterward. It is possible to get the same results with a textbook, but to do so you must be truly interested. If you understand the significance of the material you're reading and can consider how it relates to what you've learned already, you'll find yourself becoming interested and even enthusiastic. You will remember what you read with very little effort. Allow the material to make an impression on you; that is the best way to guarantee retention of it. If you treat study as a hated task, the time you spend at it will not be very productive. You must think positively and strive to enjoy what you are doing.

Some schools offer *peer tutoring,* in which more advanced students work with those who are having difficulty in their studies. The main benefit of the program is that it forces the student to pay attention to the material. Also, working with a fellow student is often more interesting and thus more meaningful than working alone. Peer tutors are frequently available at no cost or at a very reasonable cost.

A good way to help reduce wasted study time is to institute a "fine" system. After each period of study, estimate how much time you wasted with outside distractions or just daydreaming. Fine yourself for the wasted time. Pay yourself back for the time you wasted by increasing your study time requirements. A reward system is also very effective, whereby you can participate in some desired activity when your planned work or project is accomplished.

You now have a study schedule and a place for study. **TECHNIQUES** The next step is to learn proper study techniques.

I have laid out a simple four-step study plan to be used *before* the material is covered in class. There is nothing unique about this system; these general ideas have been advocated for years. One of the most important points about the study system is that you should always study prior to your class in order to obtain the maximum benefit from the class.

Step 1: Scan. Skim the text material rapidly, reading the first sentence of each paragraph. This is the quickest way to get the general gist of the material. The first sentence of a paragraph usually contains the "meat" of the paragraph, while the rest of the paragraph gives details and examples.

Step 2: Read and Question. Prior to reading the chapter, read any questions listed at the end of the chapter and objectives stated at the beginning. You'll find that the answers seem to "pop right up" as you read. After you read each paragraph, ask yourself what the paragraph actually says. Formulate an answer in your own words. Follow the same procedure as you finish each chapter.

Step 3: Recite. Read the material aloud if your study area permits. Again, ask yourself the questions that you did in Step 2. Recitation can be very effective in a group setting. The person reading can ask the others (who have each separately followed Steps 1 and 2) the questions. If for some reason you are unable to read aloud, repeat Step 2 instead.

Step 4: Refresh. Immediately prior to your class period, devote 5 to 10 minutes to a quick brush-up of your assignment.

In Step 1, pay particular attention to the author's Introduction and to the Table of Contents sections. These will give you an advance understanding of the material. Pay particular attention to conclusions or summaries to each chapter. In your reading (step 2) you will be able to understand how the author builds up to the conclusions.

Underline passages or phrases that you consider important. (A yellow accent pen also works well for this purpose.) In the margins you can put "memory joggers" — key words that tell you what a paragraph is all about. Be careful not to underline so much that your special emphasis becomes meaningless. Focus on the essential issues of each section.

Captions under pictures and diagrams are frequently very important. Also, if the author has seen fit to use boldface type or *italics,* it means that he considered the material exceptionally important.

VOCABULARY   Vocabulary is a problem area for many nursing students. Reading will not improve vocabulary unless you take the time to look up the words. However, do not look up words while you are reading, as it will completely break your concentration on the text. Underline words that you don't understand with a special color pen. After you've finished the chapter, look up the underlined words in the dictionary. Write each new word on a 3 × 5 card. Carry the cards with you and look through them when you have a few free minutes between classes or while waiting for the bus. You will quickly master the words. As you learn them, place the words in a vocabulary file to be reviewed periodically (about once a month).

Learn to recognize prefixes (such as anti-, pro-, sub-), suffixes, and word roots. An understanding of these "word building blocks" will make the task of improving your vocabulary much easier. For example, the words quadruped, orthopedic, pedometer, and pedestrian all contain the root *ped.* Once you know that *ped* means foot, you'll be able to figure out the meaning of these terms. A word with the suffix "itis" indicates infection and that with "ectomy" indicates surgical removal.

READING ASSIGNMENTS   If your instructor has given reading assignments, in addition to the text material, you should follow Steps 1 and 2 after you have completed your text reading assignment. During Step 2, take notes on any ideas not covered in the text. Include a short summary of the reading assignment (in your own words). When you are finished, ask yourself why the assignment was given. Generally, review time will not permit you to go through the reading assignments a second time, so you are going to have to rely on your notes.

Most students feel that they read too slowly and envy speed readers. Unfortunately, the claims of some speed reading courses just are not accurate. You cannot read 2000 words a minute and still comprehend perfectly what you have read. As speed increases beyond a particular point (which differs for each person), comprehension decreases.

If you have to form every word with your mouth as you read, you certainly do need help in reading. A simple aid is to clamp a pencil firmly in your mouth while you read, until you can break the habit. Another bad habit to be overcome is moving the head from side to side as you read. Your head should remain stationary; your eyes should do the moving.

Many people hear what they are reading as if they were talking to themselves. This is known as verbalizing. Even though one's lips are not moving, the verbalizing process does slow down your reading progress. Reading is a visual action; it should not be tied to an auditory process. Your school may have a remedial reading program. With help you will be able to read considerably faster than you can verbalize.

Speed in reading varies greatly, depending on familiarity with the material, the style of writing, your purpose for reading, and the difficulty of the ideas presented. For example, books that contain a great deal of scientific data or formulas take longer to read than do more descriptive texts, such as psychology books. In the next section we'll give some tips to help you to study science more effectively. When you're reading to gather data, such as to write a paper, use Step 1, the scanning process. By reading the first sentence of each paragraph you can quickly find the material that is pertinent to your needs. Many textbooks provide problems at the end of each chapter or section. The author has devised these to help you to determine whether you've fully understood the material. Do the problems on your own as best you can, without help from friends or classmates. The process of working through the problems has two major benefits: it will point out your weak areas, and it will reinforce your understanding of the material that you have mastered.

SCIENCE   Science and pharmacology present study problems for many nursing students. The basis of much of the trouble is the unusual vocabulary. Many familiar words have different meanings within a scientific field. In addition, there are a great number of unfamiliar technical words that must be learned. In addition to writing the new words on your vocabulary cards, you should also include words with which you are familiar but which have special scientific meanings.

Pay particular attention to discussions of scientific principles. Underline them (or use yellow accent pen) in your text. In addition, make out 5×7 cards for each chapter, on which you set forth the scientific principles explained in the chapter. Study these principles in the same manner as you review the vocabulary cards. Think about how each of the principles you have studied is applied.

Scientific diagrams given in the text are generally important. After studying a diagram, close your eyes and try to visualize it. If you have difficulty visualizing, attempt to reproduce the basic diagram on paper without referring to the text. When you are finished, check the text to see whether you are correct.

If you have trouble with a particular scientific concept, go to the library, where you will find other texts that cover the same material. Frequently an explanation set forth in a different manner is all that is necessary to clarify a problem.

In studying nursing and science, you are integrating many separately learned facts. Because of this, much of what you learn can be classified as "building blocks." If you don't understand the foundation material, you cannot continue with further study, as it will only confuse you. Therefore, if you are having trouble, talk to fellow students or your instructor. The longer you delay in obtaining clarification, the farther behind you will fall.

Prior to any science or nursing laboratory session, read the lab or nursing manual so that you know what will be expected of you. In your science lab, you must learn to take your time and be meticulous. Check to see that your equipment is set up properly, and, when possible, make a simple test to see that it is working properly. Follow your instructions precisely. Don't be "almost" exact. Try to be as accurate as possible with the equipment available.

Keep a notebook handy and record everything you do

in the lab and the results. Your notes will aid your memory when you review your laboratory sessions.

A great aid in nursing, science, and pharmacology courses is a thorough understanding of the metric system. Get into the habit of estimating temperatures in centigrade and converting other measurements into metric units. You will soon learn to think in metric terms.

MATH

An understanding of mathematics is important in nursing, especially in pharmacology. In computing dosages you must be accurate.

Mathematics scares many students. Actually, math simply requires you to learn a series of principles or formulas, and then to apply given facts to the proper formula. If you relate your nursing math to your daily activities of making change and writing checks, the math of computing dosages will be less frightening.

In studying mathematics, you must first read and fully understand the problem. Know what is being asked. Then make a rough estimate of the answer. If your answer differs significantly from the estimate, the chances are that either there is an error in calculations or you used a wrong formula.

Make sure that you understand why you are computing the answers in a particular manner. One way to check your comprehension is to make up a simple problem that is similar to the one you're working on. Use the mathematical formula that seems most applicable to solve the easy problem. Now apply the same principle to the more difficult problem. Your understanding of both the problem and the principle involved should be improved by this simple study aid.

The most common math errors are simple ones, such as misplaced decimal points. If you take the time to be neat, write numbers clearly, and stay within defined columns, you will significantly reduce your mathematical errors.

An important aid in studying math is to review previously learned material on a regular basis. If you are not constantly using an equation, you may quickly forget it. Budget a few minutes per week for this task and you'll have no trouble with the mathematics of nursing. In addition, your school may have a learning lab that will have many self-help math aids.

MEMORIZATION   Memorization by rote is a time-consuming and general-ly a time-wasting process. Modern education places less and less emphasis on sheer memorization. There are, how-ever, times when a list of items must be memorized in perfect order. It may also be necessary to memorize defini-tions. Memorization is a difficult task, and the longer the list to be memorized, the more difficult it becomes. There are several methods that can be used to make the process easier. Before any material is memorized, you should first understand the material fully.

Some students apply a rhythm to a list to be me-morized. They actually learn to sing the list as a tune. Chances are that you learned your ABC's in this manner, and, if asked to recite them now, you would still remember that rhythm you learned long ago.

Another method is to compose a sentence using the first letter or syllable of each word on the list to be mem-orized. Assume you had to memorize the 12 cranial nerves:

1. Olfactory
2. Optic
3. Oculomotor
4. Trochlear
5. Trigeminal
6. Abducent
7. Facial
8. Auditory
9. Glossopharyngeal
10. Vagus
11. Spinal accessory
12. Hypoglossal

The nonsense phrase "On old Olympus' towering top, a Finn and German viewed some hops" is easier for most people to remember than is the list of nerves. If you can associate each nerve to the appropriate word in the rhyme, you'll have a painless way of remembering the cranial nerves.

There are many other simple memory tricks. Suppose you had to differentiate between the terms *mydriatic* and *miotic*. Just remember that "the big word makes the pupil bigger and the small word makes the pupil smaller," and the differentiation becomes very simple. Another technique is to memorize lists alphabetically. Go through the alphabet and try to think of each word that begins with that letter.

The Bibliography lists a number of books designed to improve memory. In addition, your friends may have developed memory tricks that could be valuable to you.

LECTURES

Just before a lecture, quickly scan the material to be covered. Five minutes is normally sufficient for this process, as you want simply to refresh your memory regarding what you have learned.

In your lecture class try to find a seat directly in front of the lecturer so that you are fairly close. In this way you will be able to see blackboard diagrams and slides and to understand clearly what is said.

It is very easy to daydream when you make yourself too comfortable; you are more likely to pay attention to the instructor if you sit up straight. An attentive position is also a sign of respect for the speaker.

By looking at the lecturer's face, your hearing will actually improve, By seeing the lecturer's lips, you are more apt to hear what is said rather than what you expect to be said.

If you are overly warm it is very easy to become sleepy. Remove heavy coats and sweaters. You should not eat a heavy meal prior to a lecture, as this will make it difficult for you to remain attentive.

Don't hesitate to ask your instructor questions about statements that you don't understand. Think of the instructor as a learning resource just as books and laboratory work are sources of knowledge. Don't worry about seeming stupid. Chances are that if something is confusing to you, it is also confusing to others. However, questions of a purely personal nature and questions that digress from the material being covered are not appropriate during class time. Many instructors are glad to talk with students after class about subjects indirectly related to the lecture material. If a chemistry class arouses your interest in the news item you read this morning about the effects of artificial preservatives or of air pollution, approach your chemistry professor at the end of the lecture. Perhaps he or she can clarify some of your questions about the issues involved.

TAKING NOTES

Unfortunately, it's much easier to forget class material than to remember it. Notes are a valuable tool with which to capture your instructor's thoughts. You should have a separate notebook for each class, preferably a loose-leaf type, to which you can add or remove pages. Take notes on one side of the paper only so that your notes can be spread out for review. Each lecture should be labeled with the date and the chapter of the text being covered. In this way you will be able to study text and lecture notes together for review.

Make an effort to write legibly. Nothing is worse than trying to review lecture notes and realizing that you don't understand what your notes mean. In addition, your notes should be in your own words rather than a direct transcription of the lecture. Notes don't have to be in sentence form. A few words are adequate if they convey meaningful information.

Your notes should be clear enough so that by looking at them you can reconstruct the major points of the lecture. A simple outline format is good for note-taking. Don't try to take down everything the lecturer says. This is a common fault of inexperienced note-takers. Excessively long notes are a cumbersome review tool. Your notes should supplement the text, not replace it. Since you've already read the chapter to be discussed, you can avoid writing down material covered in the text.

In addition to notes on new material (not covered in the text), write down information that is given a different emphasis by the instructor. Another important area is any personal opinions given by the lecturer. When the speaker writes on the blackboard, it means that he or she considers the material important. This material should be set forth in your notes. Often the lecturer will tell you what is important by using phrases such as: "Be sure to note that . . . ", "the main point is . . . ", or "the real reason for . . .". You can underline or use arrows → or boxes ☐ if you want special emphasis in your notes.

Because a lecturer talks at a rate much slower than the rate which we comprehend, our minds tend to wander. The instructor might actually be saying something contrary to what we think we hear without our noticing it. This is especially likely to happen if you have a slow or uninspiring instructor.

It is difficult to listen. How often have you been introduced to a person and two minutes later you have no idea what the person's name is? You were thinking of something else, or you were not interested enough to really listen. The same tendency holds true for lectures. You spend over one quarter of your life in school. That time will be wasted if you don't make an effort to listen.

By asking yourself questions as the lecture proceeds, you can keep your attention focused on the subject. Ask yourself, "Why did he or she say that?" "How does that apply to me?" "Where is the emphasis?" However, if you take too much time reflecting on what the lecturer has said, you very well might miss an important point, so we use this technique sparingly throughout the lecture period.

Immediately after class, or as soon thereafter as possible, go over your lecture notes. If they are not clear, clarify them. Make sure that everything you feel is important is set forth in your notes.

Generally, it is not a good idea to rewrite or type your notes, since the additional benefit usually isn't worth the time spent. However, this extra step is sometimes necessary to make your notes meaningful. Notes from science classes often benefit from retyping, as do notes from any class in which the instructor is not organized and rambles. Most lecturers, however, follow a definite outline.

Some students tape lectures in lieu of taking notes. The drawback to this scheme is that tapes cannot be used readily for review because you have to listen to the whole tape, which is an extremely time-consuming endeavor. For a three-credit class, you might have over 50 hours of tapes. After all, the purpose of notes is to condense that two-hour lecture into a workable form for review, to focus on the essentials, and to have material that is in your own words.

Tapes can be valuable if you play them at times when normal study is not possible, such as when you're driving or doing your laundry or waiting for a train. Do not take your regular study time to listen to the tapes, though, because these periods can be put to better use by following the four-step study process described earlier.

When you miss a class, you have missed an opportunity to take notes. The ideal solution to this problem is to find someone who has a tape of the lecture. If you know you're going to be absent, and you have a tape recorder, ask a classmate to tape the lecture for you. If no tape is available, meet as soon as possible after the lecture with two conscientious students. Review the lecture and their notes with them. It is not enough merely to copy their notes. You must understand the instructor's emphasis and reasons for it. If the instructor is teaching several sections of a class, you may be able to make up the missed class by attending one of the other sections.

If you feel that you are not learning enough from an instructor, find out whether any other instructor is teaching the same class. Perhaps auditing another instructor's lectures will help you. You might check to see whether you can change classes. Keep in mind that a popular instructor who is entertaining is not necessarily a good instructor. Look for teachers who help their students to gain a firm grasp of the material.

You should also take notes from your lab and clinical experiences. For a science lab, write down exactly what you did and the results. For clinical lab, write down new learning experiences and patient care skills.

REVIEW

Once a week, on a regular basis, you should review all of your lecture notes from the beginning of the course up to that date. Time dulls the memory; review sharpens it. The material that is oldest, therefore, is repeated the most in review.

Study is different from review. In our studies we learn new material; in our review we are reinforcing and organizing material we have learned.

Many students who have not done their work all semester try to cram by studying blocks of previously unlearned material in a short period of time. Generally the results are not satisfactory, for the faster they try to learn, the faster they forget.

GROUP STUDY

Group study generally is not very beneficial for initial learning. Group work can, however, be very valuable for review. Learning to work with a group will be important throughout your career as a member of a health team. Group review will also help to improve your communication skills. To be worthwhile, all members of the group must have studied independently. Not much can be expected of a group that is meeting together in ignorance. One person should take charge of the review to ensure organized progression. As an example, the group could go through the lectures or clinical sessions, with one person telling what he or she considers to be the main points or ideas. Other students could supplement this with their understanding. Another valuable exercise for the group is to try to determine what questions the instructor will ask for each chapter. This is really role playing based on your experiences with the instructor.

A strong advantage of group review is that you are more likely to remain attentive when you are working with your peers, and you will thus be able to devote far more time to the subject without your mind wandering off, as is common in individual review sessions. The group forces your attention in much the same way a tutor would.

A disadvantage of a group review is that if the leader does not exercise control, it can degenerate into a "bull session" with limited benefits. Choose your group partners and leaders with care.

While you are reviewing your lecture and lab notes, you should also review the text material in order to tie the ideas or material together. A quick scan of your text should be easy, now that you have underlined important areas and added notes in the margin. If it is a laboratory course, you should of course, review your lab notes. You should also review your patient or nursing care plans as this will highlight medical therapy, diet therapy, and medications.

By learning and practicing properly planned study and review techniques, you will increase your chance for better grades as well as reduce the academic pressure of your training.

After obtaining good grades on a few tests, some students tend to feel they have it made. They find that they had studied a great deal of material that wasn't even on the examinations. They "get smart" and feel they can reduce their level of effort. They may even try to psych out the instructor and anticipate what will be on the exams, so that they can study only what is pertinent. The result of this "getting smart" is generally a significant lowering of grades. If grades are important to you, you have to keep up your study program.

NOTES

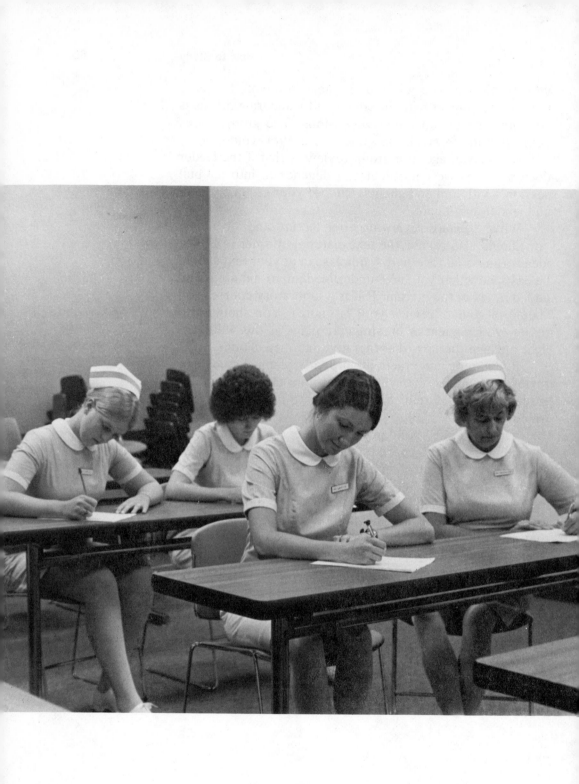

Chapter 6

How to Take an Examination

Your instructors know that examinations are not perfect measuring devices of knowledge or ability. Nevertheless, your progress in your course work will be measured by examination. While imperfect, it is the best system we have.

Look at the positive side. Treat the examination as a challenge, a chance to prove yourself. Obtaining good grades will gratify your ego and serve to increase your self-esteem. Unfortunately, all too often students view examinations negatively. You may fear failure. This fear can lead to anxiety, which can interfere with your ability to answer the questions properly. If you have done your preparation work, there is nothing more you can do. Try to relax prior to your examination. One method that helps is to sit down, close your eyes, and take 20 deep breaths. Concentrate on holding each breath for five seconds, and count the number of breaths. This exercise will help to calm your nerves; and the concentration required takes your mind off the examination. A good night's sleep before the exam will also help to reduce tension.

Most worry is unfounded. Many students worry about "horror" exams, in which they can't answer a single question. While your examination may cover an area in which you are weak, if you have studied, very few if any of the

67

questions will completely stump you. Remember that most people pass examinations.

If you mingle with other anxious students before an exam, you will heighten your own anxiety. Don't wait outside the door with the other students for the instructor to arrive. At this late time, talking to others isn't likely to help, and it is likely to confuse you and increase your nervous tension. Nervous laughter, constant chatter, and frequent trips to the washroom are symptoms of pre-exam jitters.

While you should avoid the pre-exam socializing, you do want to be close to the examination room early so you can be sure of being on time. This protects you against unforeseen delays. If you have to rush to get to your exam on time, you probably will arrive in an agitated state, and it will take some time to calm down.

When you get into the examination room, sit at your regular classroom seat if possible. Being in a very familiar position will help you to remain calm. After you start writing the examination, you will generally get so involved that any nervousness you may have will disappear.

Avoid sitting near friends. Friends can be distracting to you, and you want as few distractions as possible.

PREPARATION   Be sure to bring plenty of pens and pencils. For exams with **IBM** answer sheets, make sure you have the proper pencil (although this is usually furnished). Murphy's Law states that whatever can go wrong will go wrong; so if you have only one pen, you can count on its running dry before you finish the exam. If the examination room does not have a wall clock, a watch is essential.

If the exam calls for memorization of a list of items such as nerves or bones, write them down on the back of the blue book or a scratch sheet as soon as the test starts.

It's best to get the routine and rote necessities out of the way, to clear your mind for the questions that require your concentration. Once you actually start the test you'll be calmer than when you are waiting to start.

Some students start writing at a rapid pace as soon as the test begins. Don't do it (except to jot down memorized information). Read the instructions carefully. Read all the essay questions. Underline key words in the instructions and questions, such as "differentiate," "causes," "compare," "history," "evolution," "reasons," and "similarities." In this way you will be less likely to misinterpret the questions. On essay questions, pay particular attention to the verb. What are you being asked to do? "Compare" and "contrast" may look and sound very similar, but an essay question that asks you to compare nursing during the Civil War with nursing during World War II is very different from one that asks you to contrast them.

This preliminary reading of the questions will give you an overview of the test and the requirements. Be on your guard for unusual directions. A careful reading of the instructions might reveal that you are to answer three of the five essay questions given. If you had not paid attention to the directions, you might have given a rush treatment to all five questions rather than the detailed answers expected on just three questions.

If you're not sure what an instruction means, then by all means have your instructor clarify the meaning. You must know what is expected of you.

The instructor may also tell you how many points each part of the exam is worth. Use this information to plot the time you spend on each question. Expect multiple-choice questions (which involve reading of all the choices) to take about twice as long per question as true-false questions.

OBJECTIVE AND SUBJECTIVE EXAMINATIONS

Objective questions are true-false, multiple-choice, matching, or completion. Generally, only one answer is regarded as correct. Objective examinations are given in science and mathematics as well as in large classes, where sheer size precludes the slow grading process required with subjective tests.

Subjective examinations call for your opinions and reasoning. These consist of essay questions and are used heavily in the humanities and social sciences.

Some instructors prefer objective examinations because of the ease in grading and because they feel the measurement is more meaningful, since personal bias is eliminated. Others prefer subjective examinations because they feel this is the only way to measure the depth of your knowledge and understanding. Since the nursing state board examinations are objective, you can expect more stress on objective examinations in your nursing training.

OBJECTIVE EXAMS

Before you start on the subjective (essay) questions, which will take a great deal of time, you should first complete the objective questions, which can be answered fairly rapidly. The fact that you have them complete will also help to calm your nerves. If you do the subjective questions first and find yourself running out of time, panic could easily set in, as you would be faced with a great number of objective questions and little time in which to complete them.

From the instructions you will know whether the instructor is trying to discourage guessing. As an example, an instructor scoring a true-false exam might count the correct answers and then deduct from that score the number of wrong answers. In this case you should guess, since the odds are 50:50 for each question, even if you have no knowledge at all. Since you have studied and are prepared, you should expect to beat the mathematical odds, which represent mere chance. In addition, the methods set forth in this chapter will enable you to consistently beat the odds of pure guessing even when you are being confronted with material for the first time.

Read each question carefully and ask yourself, "What is really being asked?" Some instructors test you on the ability to read instructions and questions as well as the course material. People tend to read what they expect to see, rather than what is really there, especially when they're reading rapidly. A quick reading of an instruction such as "Which of the following is not true" could cause you to miss that all-important "not." Tests are not the place for speed reading. You must understand what is actually required.

Watch out for the "mandatory words" — always, never, and must. If there are any exceptions to the statement that uses a mandatory word, then on a true-false exam the correct answer would be "false." As an example, the question "It is good nursing practice to always have a patient deep breathe after surgery" would be false since there are exceptions. On a multiple choice question, the obvious answer might not be the correct one if there are exceptions to the statement. Questions containing mandatory words call for special care. If "balance" words such as seldom, normally, generally, and usually are used, there can be exceptions to the statement, and these few exceptions would not make the statement false. In the question given above if the word "always" were changed to "generally," then the answer would be true.

Keep in mind that even if part of a question is true, the correct answer is "false" if any part of a question is false. As an example, suppose the question were "Hemophilia is a hereditary blood disorder resulting in excessive bleeding caused by a low white blood cell count." The answer would be false, since the cause is failure of the blood to coagulate and is not caused by the white blood cell count.

Occasionally an instructor will use a double negative. If you remember that two negatives make one positive, you will not have any trouble. As an example, "least likely not to. . ." would mean "most likely to . . . ."

For multiple-choice questions you should be concerned with the best answer, not necessarily the correct answer. Don't mark down an answer until you have read all the choices. There may be several answers that are true, but one is more appropriate than the others. A careful reading of all choices may reveal that answers *a* and *c* are both correct, and that answer *d* reads "both *a* and *c*." In this case, *d* would be the correct answer.

Your instructor may include questions to test your decision-making abilities and your judgment in actual nursing situations. Draw on your experiences with patients to answer these questions.

Guessing

If you don't know an answer, you can improve your "guessing odds" by using the process of elimination. If you can discard one answer in a four-choice question as being obviously wrong, you have improved your guessing odds from 1:4 to 1:3. Of course, if you can eliminate *three* answers as being wrong, the remaining answer would have to be the correct one. Sometimes instructors throw in obviously wrong answers or even humorous wrong answers in order to complete a question. When they do this, they are really helping you by improving your odds of being right.

If you have absolutely no idea what the correct answer is to a true-false or multiple-choice question, the following simple directions will enable you to consistently beat the law of averages for guessing.

True-False Tests

1. If a question contains a mandatory word such as "always," "never," or "must," you should guess "false."

2. If a question contains a word such as "seldom," "normally," or "generally," where an exception would not alter the answer, guess "true."

Multiple Choice Tests

1. If two answers contain similar sounding words, such as "trauma" and "thrombi," choose one of these.

2. If two answers are almost identical except for a few words, choose one of these.

3. If one answer is unusually long or unusually short, choose that answer.

4. If two answers seem extreme, eliminate them. For example, if the answer choices are the numbers 3, 87, 89, and 1003, eliminate the 3 and the 1003 and take a guess at one of the two remaining choices.

5. If the question is an incomplete sentence, eliminate any answers that would create a grammatically incorrect sentence.

6. If you are unable to eliminate any answer on a four-answer question, choose the third answer. Experience has shown that it has a better than 25 per cent chance of being correct.

Changing Answers

There is a difference of opinion about whether one should change answers once they have been written. Some people feel that there is a tendency for second-choice answers to be incorrect and that it's safer to stick with your original assessment of the problem. The latest studies show that if, on reflection, you feel that an answer should be changed, you should do so. Of course, you should always change an answer when you realize that you misread a question or when another choice reveals the correct answer. Frequently you will find that questions unintentionally reveal the answers to other questions.

In taking an objective test, don't worry a question to death. Don't try to read too much into the question. Objective tests are recognition tests, so don't try to apply definitions not based on the course. Answer the questions based on your lectures and class reading, not on additional knowledge you may have. Students who have been trained in law frequently have a great deal of difficulty with objective tests because they read things into questions that the instructor never intended. Generally, your instructor will not be out to trick you, so you need not look for obscure meanings. A major fault with objective tests is that the more you know and the better you can reason things out, the more apt you are to read things into a question that were not intended by the instructor.

When questions are worth equal numbers of points, you must avoid spending a great deal of time on one or two questions. If a question requires a lengthy mathematical process, try to eliminate obvious wrong answers before beginning your calculations. If your time budget is tight, try to guess the answer to such a question. Put a star next to the answer, and go back to the question if time permits. It is much better to have made a wrong guess than to have worked it out and be right and have also left 10 questions unanswered for lack of time.

On a multiple-choice completion question, try to respond to the question in your own words without looking at the answers. Then look at the answers, and if one approximates your answer, it is likely to be the correct one.

If you have a completion question in which you cannot remember the technical word, explain your answer in your own words. You may get some credit for this, and frequently by writing down your explanation, you will think of the term.

Matching Questions

These have two columns, and you are asked to pair a word or term in one column with a word in the other. Remember that you are trying for the *most appropriate* answer. Don't assume that one answer can be used only once unless this is clearly stated in the instructions.

Never argue with the premises set forth in the question. Accept them at face value. "The moon is made of cheese and is 40 kilometers in diameter. A giant mouse can eat 100,000 cubic meters per second. How long will it take the mouse to consume the entire moon?" Don't waste valuable time being concerned that the question is not true. Guess or calculate the answer just as you would a more sensible problem.

Never add, delete, or change words in a question. If the question says "should" don't interpret it to mean "must." Read questions the way they are written and not the way you would like them to be.

Try not to skip questions. Always guess on tests that do not penalize you for wrong answers. On tests where incorrect answers are counted against you, follow your time budget based on the point value of the question. At the end of the time allotted for that question, make an educated guess if you feel that you have some understanding of the problem. The only situation in which it is appropriate to leave the answer blank is where (a) incorrect answers detract from your score and (b) you have no idea of the answer at all.

Answer Sheets

When you are answering on an IBM-type answer sheet, be careful that you are marking the correct question. If you skip a question, you may find yourself marking question 100 on the answer sheet when you are on question 99 of the test. This usually results in instant panic. Frequent checks will prevent this unpleasant situation.

Most people, when marking on an IBM sheet, blacken in the proper area by going up and down, up and down, up and down. They may use six strokes with the pencil when one would do. These few additional seconds are worth a lot more in reading the questions than in having a nice dark mark. The computer will pick up one solid mark. You will also waste a lot of time if you find that you have to erase your nice dark mark. The computer normally is programmed to indicate a wrong answer if more than one answer is marked. Therefore, you must erase completely when changing answers.

When you use a separate answer sheet, try to keep the sheet to the right of your examination (if you are right-handed). In this manner you won't have to cross over your examination to mark the answer sheet, and you will be able to keep your place on the exam and proceed faster.

SUBJECTIVE EXAMS

Objective exams require you to know certain facts; in subjective exams, you must be able to interpret those facts and to organize them into a logical statement.

Many students read the first question and immediately start to write, without much of a plan. Read all the questions and organize your first answer before you begin. Many people find that a brief outline of the points they want to discuss works well as a starting point. As you work on the first essay, ideas and information that relate to other questions will come to you. Jot these down immediately so that you can return to them at the appropriate time.

Keep in mind that your answers should be based primarily on material learned in the course. (The exceptions to this rule, as discussed earlier in this chapter, are questions that require your judgment of actual patient-care situations.) A few references to information from outside sources are acceptable; the instructor may even be pleased to see that you've done some work on your own. But the main points that you make in your essay should come from class work and not from articles you read on your own.

In answering subjective examination questions, go to the easiest question first. By completing an easy essay question, you will have more confidence because you know that you have some "guaranteed points" right at the outset.

Essays

On many essay questions it is possible to write on and on, so you must watch the clock closely. Allot a specified time for each essay, based on the point value of the question, and leave a cushion of time for a final check. When your time is up, finish your conclusion and go to the next question.

Don't start your essay by repeating the question. This simply takes time and will not give you any additional points. Think of your essay as a news story. The topics covered should include who, what, where, when, and why (the last of these is your editorial opinion). Open with your hypothesis, which is the argument you intend to prove. Your conclusion should follow naturally from the facts. If there are other possible conclusions, these should also be discussed.

The more points an essay is worth, the more carefully organized your argument should be. Certain topics are naturally suited to a particular structure. For example, essays on a history test should present information in chronological order. Think about your subject and try to determine the most logical presentation.

Remember Step 1 of the Study Process? In scanning the material, we suggested that you read the first sentence of each paragraph, because it contains the main point. Use this format in your own writing by starting each paragraph with a strong sentence. The rest of the paragraph should contain supporting data and examples.

Keep your sentences short and concise. Avoid complex sentence structure. Remember that someone has to read what you have written; the more clearly you set forth your points, generally the better will be your grade.

Don't stray from the question. Keep in mind what is being asked while you write. Remember also that you are being asked to think, not merely to list facts. Discuss data in terms of relationships, sequence of events, relevant details, possible implications, causes, examples, and other appropriate issues. The inclusion of a rough graph or table to prove a point will normally receive very favorable reaction from an instructor, as will use of the technical vocabulary of the course. If you know applicable names and dates, you should use them. In any statement or essay, the more supporting data you provide, the more valid your argument will be. Back up your opinions. Don't just state that "More people are killed with forks than with guns." Support your judgment with facts.

Organize the points you wish to make by numbering or lettering them, expanding on the rough outline you made at the beginning of the test as follows:

A high cholesterol diet can result in the following:
a.
b.
c.
d.

If you wish to call attention to a particular statement, underline it. Use of a yellow accent pen is very effective in making a point stand out. If your essay is poorly organized, and you failed to make the points in the proper order, this type of highlighting can provide a certain amount of structure.

Short paragraphs with a line left between them will make reading a lot easier for your instructor.

If a definition is asked for, you should be complete and clear. Don't give too narrow a meaning. Use the words of your instructor if possible for definitions. Your own words may not be just as good when it comes to explaining or defining.

Some teachers award high grades to dissenters who can justify their answers; others punish dissent. If you wish to take a viewpoint contrary to that covered in class, be sure to justify it. Before you offer your opinion, set forth the viewpoint of your instructor and its supporting data. This type of treatment will generally be regarded in a highly favorable light.

If you don't know the answer to an essay question, save it for last and hope that the answer comes to you as you work on the other problems. If it doesn't, and if you still have no idea what to put down, don't leave it blank.

Write about some related topic. When you are not sure, don't be too detailed; be general in your answer. Chances are you will get some credit, although not much, but this is better than zero points by leaving it unanswered. More important, once you start to write, frequently the answer will come to you. If you feel you have come up with the answer after wandering around the subject, underline the pertinent points or accent them with a yellow pen. You want to be sure your instructor doesn't overlook the fact that you finally came up with a proper answer.

Don't attempt to pad or bulk out an answer that you feel is complete. Irrelevant verbal wanderings generally detract from what you have written.

Always leave a large space between essay questions. In this way you can add to your answer later if time permits and if you think of additional points to be made. Write on one side of the paper only so that you can fill in the other side later if necessary. This applies to use of exam "blue books."

Neatness does count on a subjective examination. Instructors are going to be influenced negatively if they have difficulty interpreting what you have written.

Essays should be written in ink for ease of reading. Objective portions of exams should be written in pencil so that erasures are possible. Avoid using pencils with very hard No. 3 or 4 leads. These are not dark enough to see clearly. A No. 2 lead is recommended.

You needn't worry if some questions are longer than others. Every question will not take the same amount of time or words to answer.

Outlines

Some students have learned to answer in an outline format. As an example, suppose you were asked to explain the communication process as it relates to nursing. An outline might be as follows:

Basic Premise — Communication is an interactive process that the health-care worker uses to gather information about the patient.
I. Communication as a process
   A. Sender
   B. Receiver
   C. Message
   D. Feedback

II. When the sender is a patient there is:
  A. Connotative message
  B. Denotative message
  C. Logic and syntax
III. Nonverbal communication of the patient
  A. Congruence — the fit of the body language with the message
  B. Space and time
  C. Emotional reactions and expressions of feeling
  D. Appearance
  E. Silence
  F. Sounds — voice tone and pitch
IV. Conversation with a purpose
  A. Background in preparation for the interview as examining the charts, tests, etc.
  B. The setting
  C. Active listening
  D. Encourage conversation
  E. Insure mutual understanding
  F. Patient-centered and directed
  G. Trust

Conclusion: Communication to be effective for gathering information from the patient is an ongoing process requiring skill, experience, and evaluation.

While an outline might appear very brief, it makes your knowledge (or lack of knowledge) stand out. If you have covered the points adequately with a sentence or two of explanation for each point and example, the instructor's reaction to the outline treatment will generally be highly favorable. If you intend to use an outline format, it might be wise to ask your instructor his or her viewpoint on the use of outlines for subjective questions.

Avoid phonetic spelling and abbreviations. You might know that $\bar{s}$ means without and PSP means Problem Solving Plan, but the instructor may not understand. When the instructor doesn't understand what you are saying, your grade will suffer.

Normally every test includes something you didn't contemplate being tested on. Treat the unexpected as you would any other question. Don't panic. Rarely does one question make the difference between success and failure.

Besides the usual midterm and final examinations, your instructor may give section examinations and even unannounced or weekly quizzes. Generally, such quizzes are objective tests to make sure you are doing your required reading.

OTHER TYPES OF TESTS

Some instructors give *open-book examinations,* in which you are expected to give citations and applicable quotes. Open-book exams are usually subjective and really require the same degree of preparation as a regular examination. In order to find items quickly, color-tab your text and notebook to highlight areas you expect to find on the test. Because you can use up a lot of time looking for details or minor points, it is best to rough out the answer and then look for fill-in data as time allows.

Other instructors give *take-home examinations.* Naturally you are expected to do a much more in-depth study than for a classroom test. Your grade on this type of examination is liable to be much more critical. From a student standpoint, a take-home exam means a great deal of effort.

When you finish an examination, there is an urge to leave right away. You must fight this urge and use all of the time alloted. Proper use of this extra time can mean extra points. Go back to any questions on which you guessed at the answer. A second look at a question that stopped you the first time will frequently provide the answer. By rereading questions and answers you may find that you misread a question; or perhaps one of the other questions revealed the answer to you. Check to see that you actually wrote down everything you intended to say. Since we think much faster than we write, we often mistakenly assume that we covered a point in an essay question just because we thought of it. Check all computations and make sure decimal points are in the right place (This is the most common math error.)

AFTER THE EXAM

Don't look around when you finish to see how others are doing. All you should be interested in is yourself. In addition, looking around may give the instructor the idea that you are trying to cheat.

After you leave the class, make notes about the type of questions asked. Reconstruct the examination as best you can. This information can help you to prepare for future tests.

GRADES

The way your examination is graded will give you an indication of what the instructor was seeking. Frequently the instructor will discuss the grading system in class. If you are in doubt, even after the first examination, make an appointment with your instructor so that you can get his or her viewpoint.

Your examination results may show a need to change study and/or notetaking habits. Perhaps the instructor placed greater emphasis on clinical lab work than you anticipated. By studying the first examination, you can better know your instructor and what to expect for the next examination.

Each instructor grades subjective examinations a little differently, based on what he or she feels is important. In a study made several years ago, a large number of English teachers graded the same term paper. Grades ranged from A to D, with most of the grades in the B to C area. Obviously the paper satisfied the requirements of some instructors and failed to do so for others.

If you are able to obtain tests that your instructor used in the past, you can learn a great deal about what to expect on exams and how the questions should be answered. Some dormitories and clubs keep exam files that can give valuable insight as to what a particular instructor tends to emphasize. If your instructor is lazy, you might find questions from previous examinations repeated on your current examinations.

Grading of exams may be against a standard, such as: below 70 is a D and over 92 is an A. Grading could also be on a curve, in which a certain percentage of the class gets an A, another percentage a B, etc. When the grading is on a curve, you are really competing against your fellow students and trying to beat them to obtain a place at the top of the class. When working against a standard, you are trying for a numerical score without regard to anyone else's ability.

If you feel that your grade is unfair, make an appointment to meet the instructor. Some instructors will change a grade if you can show you really understand the material; others will not.

STATE BOARD EX-AMINATION

A major goal of your training and exams is to prepare you for your state board examination. The National League for Nursing prepares and grades these tests. The state board is a pool examination, which means that all states use the same tests. However, the passing score for the state board varies among the states.

The state board examinations are given over a two-day period. There are five sections that count for grades. Each of these sections contains approximately 150 multiple-choice questions, and the students are given two hours to complete each section. The five graded sections are Medical Nursing, Surgical Nursing, Psychiatric Nursing, Pediatric Nursing, and Obstetrical Nursing. A sixth section is included that can cover any area. It is included solely to get percentile data on new questions. After data have been gathered, decisions can be made as to whether specific new questions should be incorporated into future examinations.

Review courses for the state board exams are offered at all nursing schools. There are also many private review courses, some of which are excellent. Your nursing instructors will probably be able to suggest one of these courses if they feel it will be helpful. State board examinations for RN's are given twice a year. LPN (LVN) exams are also given twice a year, except in California, where they are given every month. Approximately 80 per cent of students pass their RN state board examination the first time.

In addition to review courses, the National Achievement Tests will prepare you for your state board exam. These tests, which are also prepared and graded by the National League for Nursing, will give each student percentile ratings with all nursing students in associate programs, diploma programs, and four-year degree programs.

The information received on your results will indicate both your strong and weak areas, which will be of tremendous aid in allocating review time for your state board.

Like the state boards, you are given two hours for each area of the National Achievement Tests.

Because of expense, most schools do not give the tests in all areas.

Tests are available in the following areas:

Anatomy and Physiology
Chemistry
Microbiology
Basic Pharmacology
Normal Nutrition
Parent-Child Care (BACC)
Medical-Surgical (BACC)
Obstetric Nursing

Nursing of Children
Psychiatric Nursing
Applied Natural Science (BACC)
Diet Therapy and Applied Nutrition
Psychiatric Nursing (BACC)
Nursing Care of Adults I
Nursing Care of Adults II
Nursing Care of Adults III
Community Health (BACC)
Natural Sciences
Maternity and Child Care
Disaster Nursing
Comprehensive Pharmacology
Basics in Nursing–DEFT
Basics in Nursing–ON
Basics in Nursing–PEN
NIP (Practical Nursing Test including pharmacology)
TUC (Practical Nursing Test on body structure, nursing, nutrition, and diet)
Mental Health Concepts
Psychiatric Nursing Concepts
Maternity Nursing for Practical Nurses
Pharmacology in Practical Nursing

There is a danger of complacency in obtaining average grades in the National Achievement Tests. Some students will take this as a sign that they will have no problem with their state boards. Overconfidence can lead to not attending school review courses as well as a cessation of study. Many students have found that overconfidence can lead to disastrous results.

However, if you have done your work and followed the advice of your instructors, you need not have any fear of examinations.

NOTES

NOTES

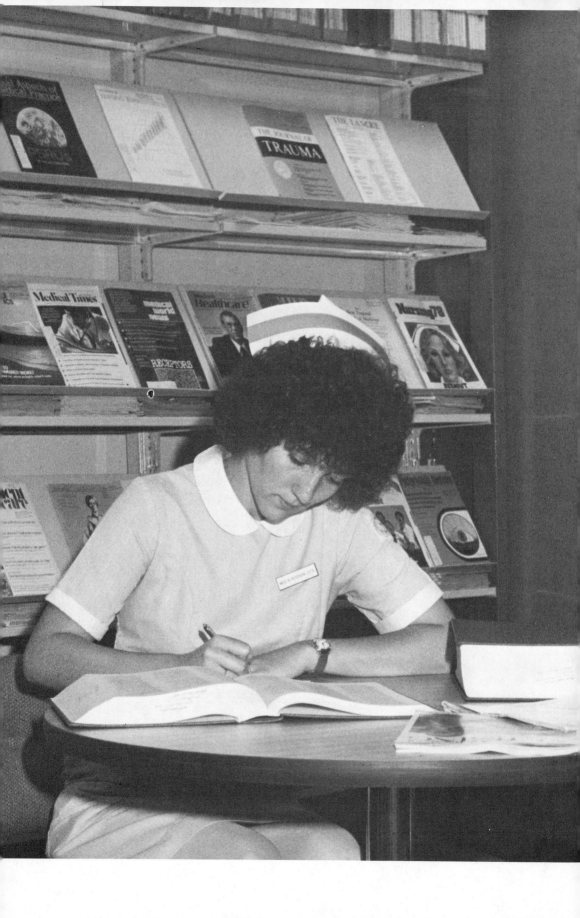

Chapter 7

Papers and Reports

Some people regard written reports as a form of medieval torture. Many students try their best to avoid certain classes just because term papers are required. Why are these projects assigned? Is it because your instructors are sadists? If you think about it for a moment, you'll see that these projects form a vital part of your education. As an educated person in our society, you must learn to express your thoughts in writing. The most effective way to develop this very important skill is to practice it. In addition, term papers provide an opportunity for you to learn outside of the classroom. Most of your formal education so far has been highly structured; you have learned what your instructors have programmed you to learn. Term papers train you to perform independent research and to evaluate facts for decision making. You are able to arrive at conclusions based solely on your own discoveries. Term papers train you to think for yourself — an essential skill for nurses.

A natural facility with words is a great help, of course, but it is far from necessary. Much more important is a well-organized plan or outline and the allowance of enough time for a thorough job. A term paper is not only a great educational experience, it can actually be a lot of fun. It is also a relatively easy way to improve your grade. And by the time you finish your paper, you'll find that your writing ability has improved greatly.

Term papers are seldom required for nursing courses. They often are assigned in elective courses, especially in the areas of psychology and sociology, and in English courses. Term papers or other lengthy reports are also required in graduate programs such as master's or doctorate degrees in nursing.

CHOOSING A TOPIC

Your instructor will probably give you some guidelines for your paper. The general area to be covered will be given fairly early during the school term. Within this area you will have to choose a specific topic for your paper. Choose a topic that is of real interest to you. Your enthusiasm for your subject will motivate you to work hard, and the result will be a high quality report.

The first place to look for a topic is your textbook. What areas related to the subject of the paper really interest you? Another source of ideas is the library. Check the general categories in the periodical index. You will find a great many specific headings that should give you some direction. The encyclopedias in your library may also provide you with an interesting subject or a unique approach to an area.

It is important to avoid an area so broad that it cannot possibly be covered or so narrow that you will have great difficulty in obtaining sufficient data. Areas that are too broad or too narrow are easily recognized by the amount of material about them in the library or the encyclopedia. A quick check of these sources will tell you that "The Renaissance" cannot be contained in a 20-page report and that it will be difficult to find enough information about "The Third Day of Millard Fillmore's Presidency" to write an acceptable term paper. You may start to prepare your paper and find that the scope needs to be limited or extended. Explain the situation to your instructor and you should have no problem in receiving approval for your revised title.

Although term papers are generally assigned for nonnursing courses, with a little imagination you may be able to find a topic that is related to nursing. A history paper, for instance, could deal with some aspect of the history of nursing. For psychology, a paper on "The Trend of Psychiatric Care for Adolescents" might be appropriate, and for your sociology term paper you could write about the sociological implications of hospitals.

Your instructor will probably give you a required number of words or pages for the report. The purpose of these guidelines is to give you some idea of the level of effort expected. The instructor is not going to count words; but he or she is going to expect your paper to be within reasonable range of the assigned length.

Talk to your friends about your choice of topics. Get opinions. You may come up with a new and fresh point of view. Ask yourself:

1. Does my topic relate directly to the assignment?
2. Will my instructor feel that the topic is a worthwhile subject?

If you are unsure about whether your subject is acceptable, discuss it with your instructor. Don't try to see the instructor before or after class, when many students are making demands on his or her time. Check office hours or make an appointment to discuss your ideas. Never come to an instructor and say, "I don't know what to write." This approach creates a very negative image. Before you meet with your instructor, follow the steps outlined thus far in the chapter — go to the library, brainstorm with friends, try to develop some preliminary ideas. Show your instructor that you are interested and concerned and that you have done some thinking on your own before coming to him or her. Most instructors are very willing to help you to develop your ideas but not to do your thinking for you. They may suggest some modification or variation of one of your ideas.

SCHEDULE

After your term paper is assigned, you should set a time table. Assume the paper is assigned September 12 and is due January 16.

Subject to be determined:	September 19
Research completed:	October 17
Rough draft:	October 24
Second draft:	November 14
Paper completed:	November 28

Only by starting to work on a term paper as soon as it is assigned can it be done in a careful manner without the pressure of unreasonable deadlines. Many students wait until two weeks (or even one night) before a report is due and then rush through it to the exclusion of their regular studies. They make the deadline, which is normally close to the date for their final exam, for which they find themselves wholly unprepared because they have been devoting time that should have been used for review to finishing their term paper. The hurried term paper is, at best, mediocre, and the final exam usually isn't any better. Remember the old story of the grasshopper and the ant? The ant, who plans for winter (which in your case is a due date and a final exam), is prepared, and the grasshopper, who chose to play during the fall, is frozen out.

RESEARCH

The first step in the research process is to make a brief outline of your paper. An outline is merely an organizational tool to help you to get your thoughts together and present them in a clear, concise order. This procedure is helpful not only for preparing material for class but also for study purposes. If you take time to think about the relationships between topics before you try to present them, you can save yourself time and frustration.

The form of an outline is designed to indicate visually the logical relationships among ideas. Begin by stating your thesis or purpose. Then list all the major divisions of supporting data, using Roman numerals. These entries should correspond to topic sentences within the proposed essay. Details within the major divisions are listed by capital letters, and further subtopics can be shown by numbered entries below the letters. For short essays, the major divisions and two or three subdivisions constitute adequate planning.

Outlines may be either by topic or by sentence. *Topic outlines* use just a few words or phrases to indicate the major and minor areas to be covered. These are sufficient for short essays, especially for those that classify or present a procedure, such as intravenous therapy. Longer essays and those papers developing a thesis can often profit from a *sentence outline*. Here you summarize, in one sentence, what you want to say about each topic or subtopic. The sentence outline forces you to formulate exactly what you want to say before you begin to write. Construction of a sentence outline allows you to test whether or not the thesis is supportable.

Consider the following examples of a sentence outline:

Thesis: We can expect hospitals of the future to dwarf our existing health care facilities.
  I. Larger facilities will reduce health care costs.
    A. They will result in greater utilization of medical and support equipment.
    B. They will allow a reduction of the ratio of administration and service personnel to medical care personnel because of better utilization of manpower.
    C. Initial per bed construction costs will be lower than for smaller facilities.
 II. Large facilities will provide better care.
    A. Greater specialization would be possible.
    B. Expensive diagnosis and treatment equipment could be provided.
    C. 24-hour laboratory and surgical facilities would be feasible.

After you've developed an outline, a good starting point for your actual research is a general encyclopedia. The library may also have specialized encyclopedias that relate to your area of study. Be sure to check with the reference librarian; don't rely on finding everything yourself. The librarian can often help you to find a variety of important reference books.

After you visit your school library, go to local hospitals and community medical societies. Often they also have libraries that contain specialized or hard-to-find material. Visit the libraries at nearby universities. Doctoral theses from the various graduate schools associated with the university are on file at the library. Use them for the valuable and often obscure material they contain and for their extensive bibliographies. A well-stocked municipal library can also be a valuable place for research. Collections vary from library to library, and your investigation of local resources will give you a sense of the scope of your school library and those in your immediate vicinity.

Note-taking is an important part of research. Many people find 5 × 7 cards to be ideal for notes. Write on one side only so they can be spread out later. On each card, indicate the source of information, listing author, publisher, title, date, and page. For periodicals (magazines, journals, newspapers), indicate title of periodical, volume, date, and page. Don't repeat similar information from different sources. You'll end up with too many 5 × 7 cards and not enough working information. When you find the same material in several books or journals, write down the full reference information for each source for inclusion in your bibliography. Look for new ideas or treatments as well as new material. Frequently you will have your own ideas about possible implications of your research. Put these ideas down on a card. Your mind is a source, as is any book or article. Remember that the purpose of research is to stimulate your own thinking.

Take notes in your own words. Don't copy what the author has said unless you intend to quote, in which case you should indicate this with quotation marks and page number. Direct quotes provide strong support for your argument. Be sure to use them sparingly, though, or their power will be diluted. Try to pick quotations that are succinct and that relate directly to the point you're trying to make.

If you find graphs or charts that you feel are valuable, make photocopies of them. Most libraries have coin-operated copying machines. Even if you don't actually include them in your report, illustrations can be useful to have in front of you while you're writing. A good chart or graph contains a great deal of information in a compact form.

Don't look only for authors who support your own point of view. Research other perspectives. After checking your textbook, the reference books, and encyclopedias, use the card files in the library. If you can't find much on your subject, look under a broader heading. If you're doing a paper on the importance of touch in nursing, you could check communication, nonverbal communication, patient relationships, etc. Books and articles on your subject often will refer to other sources in footnotes and bibliographies. These sources should also be checked.

Perhaps your best sources for research are the *Readers' Guide to Periodical Literature,* the *Index to Medical Literature,* and the *Cumulative Index to Nursing and Allied Health Literature.* However, these should be used last, after the other resources have given you a more complete foundation for this step of your research. These guides and indexes are generally multi-volume works. Start with the most current supplement. Your subject area will probably be found under much the same headings as you used in the encyclopedias. From the unbound supplements, go back year by year, taking note of the periodicals and pages you will need.

Your library may have some of the current magazines listed in the *Guides*. Most periodicals are now stored on microfilm. Your librarian will show you how to obtain the microfilm and how to use the viewer. You simply find the desired articles, read them in the viewer, and take your notes. Scan the articles on the viewer rapidly. Look for pertinent data. When you find it, read it carefully and take the necessary notes. Use the technique that you learned for your regular study projects.

Your library may not have as complete a microfilm library as you desire. A few telephone calls to other libraries in your area will tell you whether they have films you need. You may have to write directly to the publisher for some articles. Generally the publisher will either sell the back-issue to you or sell you a photocopy of the desired item.

Other sources of data are health associations and organizations. Use the *Encyclopedia of Business Information Sources* or the *Encyclopedia of Associations* (both published by Gale Research Corporation) to find applicable groups. These associations have publications and data that can be quite informative.

The *New York Times Index* may also be a good source for your research. It is similar to the periodical index except that it covers the *New York Times* only. The *Times* itself is probably available on microfilm in your school library.

If your instructor has written about your subject, be sure to pay special attention to his or her articles or books and to indicate that you have done so by footnotes and/or your bibliography.

Don't go to your instructor to say that you can't find any material about your subject. If you have carefully checked all the sources described here and have had no success, you've probably chosen a topic that is too obscure. Broaden your area of research or choose a new subject, and *then* make an appointment with your teacher to get approval for your new title. Of course, you should use your instructor as a resource if you truly have a problem.

You can readily see that research could be almost never ending, but at some time you will have to say "enough." When you find that your research has reached the point that you are simply rereading the same material in different words, you should consider calling a halt to your studies.

THE ROUGH DRAFT

Now that your research is done, you can begin a rough draft of your paper. The first step is to go through all of your note cards. Now make a new outline of your paper, since your research outline was constructed before you had any real grasp of your subject. Try to arrange your cards in accordance with the outline. Place a number on each card in sequence. (These numbers will refer you back to the source of the information for footnotes.)

It is not necessary to state, "This paper is submitted in accordance with the course requirements of. . . ." Unless a specific format is given, you should start your paper with a strong first statement that calls attention to the paper as well as sets forth your basic premise. For example:

There is nothing new about "social responsibility" or "accountability". . .we call it nursing.

Just because they call it a nursing home doesn't mean they practice nursing.

You wouldn't consciously eat garbage, but you might be better off if you did, compared to some of the "pure" food you will eat today.

Your introduction should explain the purpose or basic proposition of your paper. State how and why your thesis will be accomplished. Don't be vague. You must clearly define the subject matter of your paper.

Write the rough draft rapidly, using the 5 × 7 cards to spark ideas for you. Don't worry about style or composition at this point. Your main concern is to present the information from your notes in a logical fashion, as clearly and concisely as you can. You are not going to get by with one draft; your rough draft is a necessity. This will be your working tool to complete the paper.

Don't copy an author's words unless you want to quote. Direct quotations should be indicated. If you delete part of a quote that you feel is not needed, use ellipsis points (three dots, . . .) to show omission. Be exact. Never misquote or change a quote around for your own benefit. If you use an author's ideas, give that person credit. On the rough draft, this consists simply of a note to yourself that refers you to the proper source. Also note any sections that will require illustration.

Because you want to complete the draft in as short a time as possible, try to set aside a time period when you can devote most of a day to the task.

Attempt to show implications and give opinions as you write. Make sure you consider other ideas, if applicable, and indicate why your approach is more realistic. Avoid emotional dialogue.

You may know that AANA means Alabama Association of Nurse Anesthetists, but others may not be as well informed, so don't abbreviate. Other stylistic matters, such as the use of clichés or the overuse of adjectives, can be corrected in the final draft. The danger of using abbreviations, even in rough draft, is that you may find that you don't remember their meaning when you begin to work on the second or final draft.

After you have discussed all the data, you should have a conclusion. Your conclusion should flow naturally from the material presented. You should also consider further implications. A term paper isn't simply a conglomeration of facts. It must include your own ideas and evaluations.

When you feel the draft is finished, put it aside for a few days. When you return to it, you will probably have many new ideas and possibly even a different point of view or emphasis for your paper.

Read through your rough draft. You will find that paragraphs do not necessarily lead into each other. You will find that your organization can be improved. By cutting paragraphs out of your rough draft and putting them in a better order, using cellophane tape, you will soon have a more organized paper. After you have reorganized your rough draft, and possibly made notes for changes, you should start writing your second draft.

THE SECOND DRAFT

On your second draft you can take your time. Make sure that each paragraph reads properly. Now is the time to begin to polish your writing style. A simple, direct tone is most appropriate for research papers. Avoid dramatic phrases with lots of unnecessary adjectives. Extravagant writing is fine for advertising copy but has no place in nonfiction. On the other hand, try not to use the same word or phrase more than once every few paragraphs. Repetition detracts from the meaning of a term and is boring to the reader. Use a thesaurus or a dictionary of synonyms and antonyms to find a variety of words that have similar meanings. For instance, when you look up "implication" in a thesaurus, you find that "connotation," "inference," "supposition," and "significance" may be substituted for it, depending on the context.

Clichés such as "hard as nails" and "smooth as silk" should never be used in any kind of writing. They have been heard so often that they no longer have any power; people use clichés only when they're too lazy to create an original way of expressing themselves.

As you read each sentence, ask yourself whether you could make your point more clearly. Put yourself in the reader's place. In this case, the reader is your instructor, and he or she has a great many term papers to read. Try to write in a style that you would find lively and interesting if you were the teacher.

Each paragraph should start with a sentence that sets forth the main point of the section. The rest of the paragraph should contain supporting detail. In addition to being easy to read, this format helps your instructor in grading, since often, when a large number of papers are turned in, an instructor will read the first sentence of each paragraph and then go to the supporting detail only when of special interest. Avoid overly long paragraphs. Short paragraphs make material easy to read.

Don't try to impress the instructor with your great learning. Use simple English except when dealing with technical terms. If an explanation of a term is necessary, make sure it is included. Don't pad your paper with words to reach a desired number of pages. Padding usually detracts from what you are saying.

As you prepare your second draft, ask yourself the following questions:

1. Does my work reflect the level of effort expected by the instructor?

2. If I knew nothing about the subject, would I be led to the stated conclusions?

3. Does my paper appear to follow all specific instructions given?

The second draft, in some instances, can be the final copy, but don't count on it. It may need corrections or a complete revision. Also, your final draft should be neatly typed. Handwritten papers are difficult and, in many cases, nearly impossible to read. On an examination, some sloppiness and grammatical errors are expected; on a term paper they are not acceptable.

It is very difficult to proofread your own copy, as you tend to read what you expect to find rather than what actually appears. Have a friend proofread for continuity, clarity, grammar, spelling, and punctuation. After proofreading, you are probably ready for typing.

THE FINAL DRAFT: FORM AND CONTENT

Use 8½ × 11 inch white bond paper. Pica type is preferable to the smaller elite or the fancy script type, both of which are difficult to read.

Your *title page* should indicate the name of your school, the title of the article, the course name and number, the section number, instructor, and, of course, your name. A sample title page follows:

W H Y H E L P?
by Francis Roberts
Podunk City College
Nursing 101
Section 3
Instructor: Hubert Cummings

In the event you are given a specific format for the cover page, you should, of course, use it.

The title of your paper should tell something about your paper and catch the interest of the reader. Catchy titles sell commercial products and can help your paper. Bear in mind, however, that your primary objective is to convey information. A too-cute title that explains nothing is of no value.

Your final typed copy should have a two-inch lefthand margin to provide space for the instructor's comments. It should be double spaced, and all quotes should be indented or be set off by quotation marks. Quotations may be single spaced.

Number each page. It is best to indicate "page 1 of 12," "page 2 of l2," etc., and to include your name at the top of each page. In this way, pages will not get lost or out of order.

Footnotes are used to tell the reader where you obtained your information.[1] Not all types of data require footnotes; of course, if they did, you'd have to supply a footnote for every sentence! Only material that is original to the source from which you obtained it should be footnoted. For example, it is not necessary to provide a footnote for the statement that Columbus discovered America in 1492. This known fact, which is easily available in numerous books, is considered general knowledge. If you read a study of early explorers to the New World, in which the author did her own research, uncovered new facts, and formulated an original hypothesis from those facts, you would provide a footnote identifying this author in your discussion of her theory.

Indicate footnotes with numbers placed above and to the right of the appropriate word. Use Arabic numbers, and number consecutively. Place footnote references at the bottom of each page or at the end of the paper.[2]

Footnotes for books should show all the reference information listed on your 5 × 7 cards — author, title, publisher, place of publication, year of publication, and page. The title should be underlined. A typical reference footnote would look like this:

[27]William Pivar, *Getting Started* (San Francisco, CA.: Canfield Press, 1976), p. 93

The footnote style for magazines is as follows:

Healthcare — *Children in Trouble,* Vol. XXV, Sept. 14, 1968, pp. 29–30

The term *ibid* is used for a footnote source identical to the one preceding it. If the page number is different, you should list it:

Pivar, *ibid.,* p. 27

Details of proper organization and footnoting are described in *A Manual for the Writers of Term Papers, Theses and Dissertations* by Kate L. Turabian. This short book,

---

[1]Footnotes are also used by many authors for statements that are interesting or important but that are not directly relevant to the main focus of the discussion. You will not be using footnotes for this purpose in your term paper, but you may see them used this way in your research, and you should be aware of this other function.

[2]For term papers, footnotes are usually placed at the end of the paper rather than at the bottom of the page.

published by the University of Chicago Press, is available in paperback.

Find out whether your school has a particular format for footnotes and whether your instructor has a preferred style, and follow the instructions as given.

Mount any graphs or pictures firmly on 8½ × 11 inch paper. For more attractive lettering on graphs or title pages, you might consider press-on black letters, available at most stationery stores. Graphs should be done in black ink for clarity. They should be dark enough so that they can be photocopied if necessary.

At the end of your paper include a complete bibliography, listing sources in alphabetical order by author. The listings in the bibliography should follow the same format as the footnotes. Go through your 5 × 7 cards and cite all the sources that you read, including those that do not appear in the footnotes. One purpose of the bibliography is to provide research information for other readers who may want to read more about your topic on their own, just as you used bibliographies of other books in your research. In addition, the bibliography shows the teacher how much research you have done beyond the sources that you listed in your footnotes. Instructors are impressed by lengthy bibliographies that indicate a great deal of research, but they are rarely fooled by excessively long lists or fake sources. Many will check entries that sound doubtful. If you've done enough research to write a creditable report, your bibliography will be fine; don't detract from an otherwise good paper by tacking on an unrealistic or unbelievable list of reference sources.

To make your paper look better and to show your pride in your accomplishment, you can back it with a blue legal backing, available at most stationers, or use a cardboard or plastic binding, available at your bookstore.

Don't try to use someone else's work as your own. *Plagiarism* is the theft of someone else's efforts, and an act of this type will raise a question as to whether you have the proper moral character for the nursing profession. Most instructors can spot plagiarized material readily because the organization and grammar are different from (and often better than) your own. It is common for instructors to come across papers that they know they have read before. It usually doesn't take too much effort to find out where, and the result is disastrous. Even though many fraternities and sororities have term paper files, using them for anything other than research is like playing Russian roulette. Even if you are not caught, the grade you get may not really be that good, and you certainly will not have learned anything.

NURSING HISTORIES

In nursing you will be expected to write nursing histories and care plans. Nursing histories contain information received from records and discussion with the patient. In preparing nursing histories you must learn to listen and ask questions for clarification. A nursing history is the first step in planning effective nursing care. From the nursing history a written care plan is formulated. Every institution has a different format for nursing histories, but in all cases it is essential that the history be complete. Some nurses prepare their own checklists so that they are sure that all pertinent areas have been covered.

CARE PLANS

A care plan is a comprehensive report about a patient. It enables the staff to provide the patient with the kind of care that the patient has a right to expect.

The purposes of nursing care plans are:

1. To provide individualized information.
2. To help in setting priorities. Immediate patient needs and problems are attended to first.
3. To provide a means of systematic communication among members of the health team and to coordinate the various aspects of treatment.
4. To provide continuity to the nursing care process.
5. To assist in evaluating the care actually provided.
6. To provide a continuous nursing learning tool.

A care plan should take in the psycho-social aspects of the patient's well-being as well as physical problems. It should be complete so that a reader will fully understand the patient's situation and know how to intervene. Your school probably has a suggested format for care plans. Regardless of the structure, what is essential is that your care plan be concise yet complete statements that indicate the conditions and the extent of the required action. Care plans should include brief statements of measurable patient goals. Samples are given on the next three pages.

SAMPLE

GENERAL NURSING HISTORY
NURSE'S ADMISSION NOTES

Date_____Time_____Room_____Age_____Sex_____|

Mode of Admission_____|

Accompanied by_____   Reason for admission_____

TPR:_____ BP:_____HT:_____WT:_____

Allergies: Drug_____   _____
        Food_____
        Other_____   Patient perception of illness_____
Dentures: Upper_____Lower_____Partial_____   _____
Eyeglasses_____Contacts_____Prosthesis_____
Valuables (describe) Watch_____   Previous hospitalization: When_____
        Rings_____   Where_____
        Other_____   Reason_____
        Disposition_____
                      Chronic illnesses_____How long_____
Orientation to room: Call bell____ Bed Op_____   Diabetes_____   _____
    Roommate__ _____Clothing storage_____   Cardiac_____   _____
                         Other_____   _____
    Signature_____   _____   _____
                         _____   _____

NURSING ASSESSMENT: Medications: (dosage and frequency included)
    Date_____Time_____   _____
                         _____
Mental status_____   _____
                         _____
Senses: Hearing_____Vision_____   Disposition of Meds_____
        Other_____
                         Food habits
Ambulatory ability_____   Diet_____
                           Beverage_____
Skin condition_____   Alcohol Usage_____
                           Freq. of meals_____
Emotional status_____   Sleep patterns_____
                           Get up_____
Physical disabilities_____   Bedtime_____
                           Other_____
Other_____   Elimination pattern_____
_____   Bowel_____
_____   Bladder_____
_____   Bath Pattern_____

History relevant to present illness_____
_____
_____
_____

Other observations and comments_____

Routine: Lab_____X-ray_____

                    Nurse's Signature_____
Figure 7–A

SAMPLE

PEDIATRIC NURSING HISTORY

Up to 12 Months
PATIENT INFORMATION

Informant_____ Date_____ Time_____

Admitted per Ambulatory_____ Armband on Patient_____
             Wheelchair_____ Name on Wall Plate_____
             Stretcher_____ Accompanied By_____

B/P_____ (L,R)   Prosthesis_____ Dentures_____

Temp._____ (O,AX, R)   Valuables_____ Urine Specimen_____

Resp._____ (Normal – Difficult)

Pulse_____ (reg., irreg.)

Names and ages of other children in family? _____

Have you ever been hospitalized before? _____ why? _____

Is child on any medication? _____

Does someone plan to stay with child? _____
_____

| Eating Habits |

Breast fed_____ uses bottle_____ spoon_____
cup_____ Holds bottle_____ Present formula_____
Feeding schedules_____ Food likes_____ dislikes_____
Juices_____

| Sleep Habits |

Bedtime_____ crib_____ regular bed_____
Does child sleep alone? _____ light on or off_____
Does bed have sides?_____
Does child sleep with anything special? _____

| Play Habits |

Favorite toy_____ Plays alone or with other children_____
grownups_____

| Physical Abilities |

Walks_____ with help_____ Holds head erect_____
Sits up_____ Stands_____ Crawls_____
Follows objects with eyes_____ Holds objects_____
Shows preference for which hand?_____

| Socialization |

Responds to smile _____
Pays attention to spoken word_____
Responds to name_____
What words used for Mother/Father? _____

| Hygiene |

What is used for child's bath? sink_____ basin_____
sponge_____

Figure 7–B

What kind of soap is used?_____ lotion_____ oil_____
powder_____
What do you use for diaper rash? _____
What detergent do you use for baby diapers? _____
Do you use bubble bath?_____

Comments   Nursing Observations

_____   _____
_____   _____
_____   _____
_____   _____

Figure 7–B *Continued*

NURSING CARE PLAN	
NURSING PROBLEMS AND NEEDS	PLAN OF APPROACH

ORDER DATE	MEDICATION	STOP DATE	ORDER DATE	MEDICATION	STOP DATE

SURGERY DATE	DIAGNOSIS	IN CASE OF EMERGENCY NOTIFY		SPECIAL INSTRUCTIONS	
TYPE OF SURGERY		RELATION-SHIP	PHONE		
		RELIGION	LANGUAGE SPOKEN		
NAME	ROOM NO.	ADMISSION NO.	PHYSICIAN	ADMISSION DATE	AGE

Figure 7–C. (Courtesy of Physician's Record Co., Berwyn, Illinois.)

OTHER PAPERS AND REPORTS

You may be assigned other reports or reviews. A report is a paper based on your own work; a review is normally a critical evaluation of someone else's work.

For a *book report,* briefly describe the contents of each chapter. State the author's moral or theme and its relevance to the world as you see it. Discuss your agreement or disagreement with the author's ideas, giving reasons for your beliefs. In writing a book report, you should consider why the report was assigned. Does the instructor want you to provide an in-depth analysis of the historical or social significance of the work? This is often the teacher's reason for assigning a report on a classic author such as Shakespeare. Is the instructor looking for your judgment of the morals or ethical position taken by the author? In this case, you should be sure to describe fully the moral viewpoint of the author as you see it before discussing your reaction to it. Perhaps the purpose of the report is to compare a book with other works that you read for the course. If you're not sure why a book has been assigned, meet with the instructor or your classmates to get a clearer idea before you begin to struggle with an assignment that you don't understand.

Some instructors ask students to make a separate oral report. Sometimes these are in connection with term papers. For an oral report, as with your term paper assignments, choose a subject in which you are interested. You are more likely to be enthusiastic in your presentation of a topic that fascinates you. Start your report with a strong statement to get immediate attention. State your purpose, give supporting evidence, and then tie everything together with a conclusion. Follow the same steps that you took in preparing your written report.

Of course, the main difference between an oral and a written report is that you must stand up in front of a group to present your oral report. The prospect of presenting an oral report makes many students nervous. Some students avoid classes for which oral reports are required. It is natural to be nervous when you know that you are going to be graded on a presentation and that a large number of people will be watching and listening to you. But once you start, your tension will lessen significantly and in many cases will disappear completely before the report is finished.

Practice presenting your report in front of a mirror. Try to vary your voice inflections. Speaking in a monotone is the fastest way to put your listeners to sleep. Try for eye contact with your audience. Use cue cards with key words or phrases to jog your memory. In this way, you won't have to read the report, and it will sound much more natural. Ask a friend to listen to you and evaluate your report. Often someone else can be a great help in pointing out areas that need clarification or areas of omission.

After a clinical experience the clinical group will meet. You will be expected to relate the clinical learning to class learning and patient care.

No matter what kind of report you give, you should learn to plan. The phrase "The early bird catches the worm" does apply, especially when the worm is really good grades.

NOTES

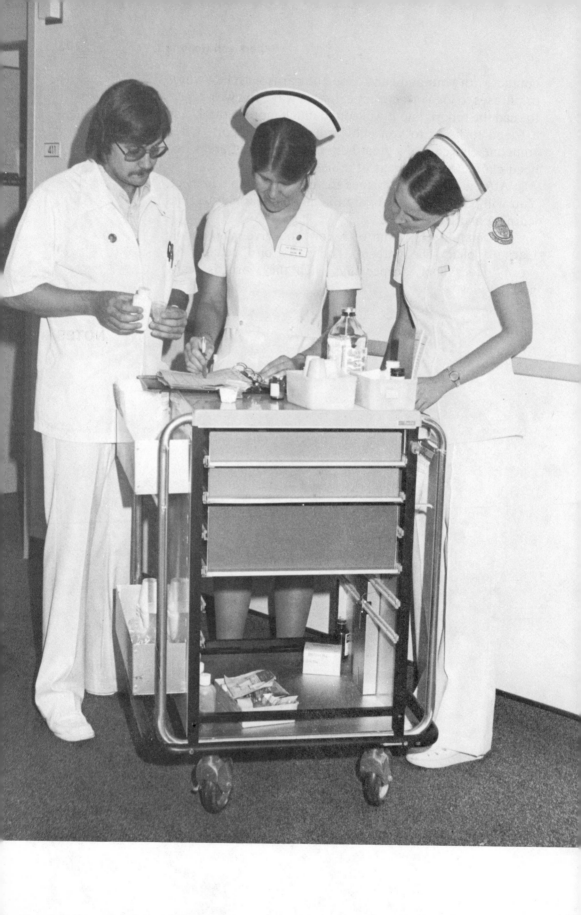

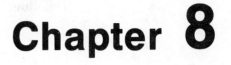

Chapter 8

Financing Your Education

The best things in life don't seem to be free when you start planning your finances for your nursing education. You will have to consider expenses such as:

Tuition
Room and board
Books
Transportation
Insurance
Clothes (including uniforms)
Nursing equipment (watch, scissors, stethoscope, etc.)
Laundry and cleaning
Entertainment and recreation
Miscellaneous

Ideally, financial planning for your education should begin well before you enroll in a nursing program. Educational costs, like everything else, have increased with inflation. Some schools are now charging over $6000 per year just for tuition and room and board. Because of continuing cost increases, you can expect your expenses during your last year to be greater than first year expenses. For planning purposes you should estimate at least a 6 percent increase in costs each year.

The three basic solutions to any financial problem are:

1. Increase income
2. Lower expenses
3. Go into debt

All three of these possibilities will be considered in this chapter.

INCREASING YOUR INCOME

Scholarships

One way to increase your income is to obtain a grant or scholarship. There are many thousands of scholarships available, ranging from very small amounts to full four-year scholarships.

Information about local scholarships can be obtained from your guidance counselor or your financial aid office. You will find that there are many scholarships specifically for nursing students, such as those offered by professional nursing groups.

National scholarships and other forms of financial assistance are described in the booklet "Scholarships and Loans for Beginning Education in Nursing," available at a small charge from the National League for Nursing, 10 Columbus Circle, New York, New York 10019. Three excellent books about scholarships are *How to Get Money for College* by Benjamin Fine and Sidney Eisenberg, *College Scholarship Guide* by Clarence E. Lovejoy and Theodore Jones, and *Lovejoy's College Guide*.

The American Legion publishes a booklet entitled "Need A Lift," which includes sources of loans and scholarships as well as career guidance information. The booklet is available from the The American Legion Education and Scholarship Program, Americanism and Children and Youth Division, Indianapolis, Indiana 64206.

The American Medical Association publishes a Financial Information National Directory (FIND). This 300 page directory lists more than 1000 sources for financial assistance for medical studies, including nursing. It is available for $2.95 from the A.M.A., 535 North Dearborn, Chicago, Illinois.

For minority students a booklet entitled "Going Right On" is available without charge from the College Entrance Examination Board, Publications Office, Box 592, Princeton, New Jersey 08540.

ASPIRA is an agency for helping Puerto Rican students. Write Aspira, College Retention Counseling, 216 West 14th Street, New York, New York 10011.

The Association for Chicanos for Admissions provides financial aid for Spanish surnamed students. Write P. O. Box 604, Ypsilanti, Michigan 48196.

The National Chicano Health Organization aids Chicano students in the health education area. Their address is 1709 West 8th Street, Suite 807, Los Angeles, California 90017.

"Mas Education. . . Mas Oportunidad" outlines opportunities for Spanish speaking youths. It is available from the U. S. Department of Health, Education and Welfare, Washington, D. C. 20202.

"Scholarships for American Indians" is available from the Bureau of Indian Affairs, Branch of Higher Education, 123 4th Street, S. W., P. O. Box 1788, Albuquerque, New Mexico 87103.

"Health Careers for American Indians and Alaska Natives" covers financial assistance. It is available from the Indian Health Service, Health Service and Mental Health Administration, Public Health Service, U. S. Department of Health, Education and Welfare, Rockville, Maryland 20852.

The National Scholarship Service and Fund for Negro Students offers supplementary scholarships. For information write 1776 Broadway, New York, New York 10019.

Most institutions require you to fill out either a PCS (Parent's Confidential Statement) or an FFS (Family Financial Statement) if you apply for financial aid. If you (a) received less than $600 from your parents in the past year, (b) have lived away from home at least a year, and (c) are not listed as a dependent by your parents for tax purposes, you will be required to fill out an SFS (Student Financial Statement). Information for these forms can be obtained from tax returns.

Since aid is generally based on need, a need analysis will be made by the school. Your need represents the difference between the amount determined to be your estimated expenses and what, based on the financial reports, your family can contribute.

Many schools offer aid packages that are combinations of scholarships, grants, loans, and jobs. Often the scholarship consists of a reduction in tuition.

Most people have exaggerated ideas about the amount

of scholarship money that is available. While you should definitely apply for every scholarship for which you qualify, you should not base your decisions to continue your training solely on whether or not a scholarship is received. This is particularly true for students from middle income families. Today, many scholarships are based wholly or partially on financial need rather than solely on academic standing. If your parents are above the poverty level, it is difficult to obtain a substantial scholarship.

If you can show the need, one particular grant that is available is the Basic Educational Opportunity Grant (BEOG). This is a federal aid program, and unlike a loan, it need not be paid back. Awards are based on need and are given to undergraduate students. The grants range from $200 to approximately $1600 and are intended to help meet educational costs. For applications and information about basic grants, see your financial aid office or write Basic Grants, Department of Health, Education and Welfare, Office of Education, Washington, D. C. 20202.

Students from extremely low-income families can also qualify for Supplemental Educational Opportunity Grants (SEOG). Money is allocated to participating schools for this program from the Department of Health, Education and Welfare. For information on eligibility and availability of funds you should see your school's financial aids officer.

The federal government has a program specifically for nursing students, The Nursing Student Loan and Scholarship Program. Information as to this program can be obtained from your school's financial aids office.

The scholarship portion of the program is for full- or half-time students in good standing. Scholarships are for a maximum of $2000 per year or the amount of the student's need, whichever is less. If you're enrolled in a full 12-month program, the maximum increases to $2667. Scholarship awards are, of course, similar to grants in that they need not be paid back.

You should also talk to your instructors or advisors about available scholarships. Frequently they can help you to obtain one.

Jobs

A full- or part-time job is the most common form of financial aid. However, nursing is a demanding course of study, and few are able to work full-time and continue their nursing training.

Most students can at least work part-time and during summer vacation. An average student should be able to earn around $2000 per year without jeopardizing grades.

A job that relates directly to your nursing career goal is, of course, the most desirable type. Chapter 10 deals in large part with obtaining this type of job.

Other jobs that are particularly attractive to students are waiter and waitress jobs in supper clubs. Little training is needed, the hours are compatible with your schedule, the income (because of tips) is above average, and meals are generally included. In addition, restaurant jobs are available on a regular basis because of the high turnover of employees within the field. It may, however, be necessary to start at a position clearing tables or cleaning and to move gradually up to a waiter or waitress position.

Other desirable jobs for students are as car parking attendants at clubs and restaurants, and as tutors for college, high school, or grammar school students.

There are many jobs available that offer room and board, such as caring for a child as a babysitter or governess, companion or aide for the elderly, or chauffeur. Nursing students are in demand for these types of jobs. Although these positions do not always include a salary, they generally do not require a great many hours. They are also relatively easy to obtain. Contacting home health agencies and nurse registries is normally effective.

Your student employment office, as well as your state employment office, can help you find a job; however, you should be aware that employers who contact these sources are frequently looking for cheap labor.

Some jobs, such as late night desk duty at a convalescent home, pay very little but offer an opportunity to study when you are not busy.

If it is necessary to earn the maximum amount during the summer, you should consider work in the construction industry. If you can obtain one of these positions, you can expect to do well, because of high union wages. In recent years, women have been employed as flag persons on many road jobs.

One unusual problem for students has been that of getting too good a job. An excellent position can be a temptation to quit school. While it may not necessarily be a wrong decision, you should be certain it is well thought out and not simply used as an excuse to leave school.

Some schools offer *work experience programs*. These

are generally classified as parallel or alternate plans. In a parallel program, the student works while going to school. The student obtains some college credit for working and usually completes some work-related project.

In the alternate work experience program, the college usually sends a small group of students to a job in their career field. The students then alternate between going to school full-time for a term and working full-time for a term. While it takes twice as long to finish your training under the alternate program, you are able to save enough during each work period to pay the expenses for the next school period. The work experience administrator at your school may be able to place you in a position for either the parallel or the alternate program.

At times the Armed Services have had programs for the professional education of nurses. At the present time, because of funding restrictions, none of these programs are available. Check with your guidance counselor to find out whether this service is reactivated.

R.O.T.C. training is available for nursing students enrolled in bachelor degree programs. During the 3rd and 4th year the student receives $100 per month from the government. The program *does* requires a service commitment. Details of these programs are available from your campus R.O.T.C. office.

Parents

You should sit down with your family to find out what financial commitment they can make. They should have a realistic idea of the total educational costs based on present and anticipated expenses. In the event that they decide that they can pick up all the expenses, you should consider yourself lucky. At the other extreme, they may decide they can't help you at all, in which case you will be on your own. They may decide they can pay tuition only, or tuition and dormitory room and board costs, or simply a given amount of money per year. Your family will have to analyze their ability to help based on their income, other financial commitments, expenses, and savings.

A form of savings frequently overlooked by parents or spouses are life insurance policies. It is possible to borrow on these policies at comparatively low interest rates. Life insurance has sent thousands of students through school. Sometimes parents obtain loans from banks, credit unions, or even relatives, to finance their children's education.

Because of inflation, if your family owns a home there is probably a substantial equity. Refinancing or taking a second mortgage can be a means of raising money.

The final decision should be based on realistic cost estimates and careful evaluation of financial status. Frequently in large families, even those with substantial incomes, the parents' aid to each child will, by necessity, be limited.

Marriage before graduation frequently increases financial problems. Some parents use it as an excuse to stop or reduce the aid to a son or daughter. They may say, "If you're old enough to marry, you're old enough to take care of yourself." By talking to both sets of parents in advance, it may be possible to continue educational support for both you and your spouse.

If one of your parents is receiving Social Security benefits or is deceased but was covered by Social Security, you are probably eligible for Social Security educational benefits. To receive these benefits you must be a full-time student. Check with your local Social Security office as to your eligibility. The War Orphans Educational Act provides benefits for children of totally disabled veterans and those whose parents died from service-connected disability.

Some colleges and institutions offer half-time nursing training. This allows you to work while in the program. Of course your training will take longer than if you were a full-time student.

LOWERING YOUR EXPENSES

One way to lower expenses is to reduce your time in school. By carrying course overloads and/or attending summer sessions (if you are on a baccalaureate program), it is possible to complete a four-year nursing program in three years.

In some families where there are several children close in age, the children take turns going to school. The parents support only one child at a time. In the same way, many husbands and wives take turns, with the husband getting the degree while the wife works, and then working in turn while the wife finishes school.

Expenses and Saving

Ben Franklin was right when he said that "a penny saved is a penny earned." Cutting school expenses by $1000 per year is the equivalent of earning $1000. One way *not* to save money is by sharing *books*. Grades are too important to have to rely on the availability of a shared book.

By buying used textbooks directly from other students, you can save significantly on your book expenses. Your bulletin boards usually list many used books for sale. You can often buy used books at half price. In addition, many bookstores in college areas, as well as school bookstores, carry used texts at approximately 1/3 off the new price. Because of the demand for used books, you should try to buy them as soon as you know you are registered in a class. Make sure the used book you are buying is both the proper text and the current edition for the required class.

Clothing can be a major expense or a minor one. Today student fashions are much more casual. You can outfit yourself satisfactorily from Brooks Brothers on the one hand or the Salvation Army store on the other. Because styles vary at different schools, don't buy an extensive wardrobe prior to attending school. First year students tend to be the most fashion conscious students. After the first year, students tend to show more individuality in dress.

You will need uniforms. Each school has its own uniform requirements. Usually three complete uniforms and one good pair of shoes are necessary. You should buy good quality wash-and-wear uniforms that will wear well and drip dry.

Room and board is a major area of expense. If your school maintains dormitories, you will find that, generally, this is the most economical housing available. Occasionally, by sharing an apartment with several students, you can obtain lower overall costs.

Rent is a variable cost, and savings are possible. A room can usually be rented for much less than an apartment. With a room you will have to buy meals as opposed to an apartment, where you can cook. Nevertheless, an apartment is generally more costly. If you share an apartment, you can reduce costs significantly.

While *food* costs can be cut, you should keep in mind that nursing is hard work, and you must keep yourself physically fit. A breakfast including milk and eggs will provide you with energy and "brain power" to start the day. In your nursing training you learn the importance of a well-balanced diet, including meat, vegetables, fruit, cereal, and milk products. Fad diets should be avoided, as they generally lack basic nutritional requirements for maintenance of good health.

Of course, if you can live at home throughout your training you will have significantly reduced costs. Sometimes it is possible to live with relatives in the area.

Many students work for their meals at sorority or fraternity houses or at local restaurants. Frequently you can arrange to work one hour in exchange for a meal.

Laundry and cleaning expenses can be cut down by use of laundromats and cleaning machines. Many students have a travel iron to keep their wardrobe in good shape.

Today one of your largest expenses will be your *car*. When confronted with a choice of continuing school or keeping their car, students often choose their car instead of their education. Our society places a great deal of importance on owning a car, and the need for private transportation is great for many people. However, there are many viable alternatives to owning a car. Public transportation, motorcycles, bicycles, walking, and friends with cars should all be considered. Car repairs, payments, parking fees, oil and gas, and insurance can exceed room and board expenses. In some situations, a car is a necessity; more often it is a luxury. It is frequently more economical to rent a car when one is absolutely essential than to endure all the expenses of ownership.

You should, whenever possible, avoid long-term *financial obligations*. Buying things on installment credit, even if it means only a few dollars per month, can turn into a burden when you find yourself counting pennies. Similarly, you should avoid long-term commitments such as apartment leases. It might seem like a good idea for you and two other students to sign a one-year lease for an apartment, but you might find yourself obligated for the entire rent should you lose your roommates. Whenever possible, a month-to-month rental is preferable.

Avoid signing any document that can possibly lead to future financial obligations. As an example, you should never cosign for anyone else on a loan unless you are able and willing to pay that person's debt. All too often the cosigner ends up paying.

Some additional ways to save money are:

1. Make out a budget. Study your checkbook to get an idea of where your money goes. Strive to live within the budget.

2. Don't change your spending habits on pay day or whenever you receive money. Frequently students tend to purchase more non-necessities during these periods.

3. Carry only a minimum amount of cash with you. This reduces your ability to spend impulsively for non-necessities.

4. Use checks only for paying bills or emergencies. Because checks are not like "real money" too many people tend to spend more with checks than they would with cash.

5. Do not use credit cards. They are an easy way to upset your budget. People spend more freely with credit cards than they do with cash.

6. Make a shopping list of what you need. Buy only what is on the list. This is to avoid impulse spending for wants rather than needs.

7. Avoid rationalizing small expenses when "it's only a dollar" or "for five dollars you can't go wrong." Ask yourself, "What would happen if I didn't buy?"

LOANS

The third alternative to financial problems is to go into debt. While you might have difficulty borrowing money, your parents, by cosigning, can help you to borrow money even if they are unable to help you directly.

Check with your financial aid office. Many schools have student loan funds for both regular aid and emergency aid. In addition, many states provide special student loan programs.

The Nursing Student loan program is available for full- or half-time nursing students in good standing. The student must shown financial need and cannot have a concurrent loan from the National Direct Student loan fund. The loans are up to $2500 or the amount of the student's need, whichever is less for each academic year. If the school is on a 12-month basis rather than the traditional 9 months, the loan can be increased to $3333. The total federal loans to any student cannot exceed $10,000.

A unique aspect of the Nursing Student loan is that the student may be eligible for cancellation of a portion of the loan. After being licensed as an R.N., if you are employed by an approved public or *nonprofit* private agency, institution, or organization, the rate of cancellation of the loan is 15 percent for the 1st, 2nd and 3rd year of such service and 20 percent for the 4th and 5th year. A total of 85 percent cancellation including interest is therefore possible.

If you are interested in continuing your education beyond an R.N., there are many programs available to help you.

The Professional Nurse Traineeships program of 1956 has been extended. It awards long-term traineeship positions to R.N.'s for advanced education in administrative, supervisory, or clinical specialization. There is even a program for baccalaureate degree preparation for R.N.'s with an AA degree or a diploma.

The Children's Bureau of the Department of Health, Education and Welfare gives fellowships for advanced study in maternal and pediatric nursing.

The Rehabilitation Services Administration of the Department of Health, Education and Welfare provides traineeships to graduate nurses to increase the supply of nurses to administer or teach rehabilitative nursing to physically or mentally handicapped persons.

The National Institute of Mental Health has a financial assistance program to further education of psychiatric and mental health nurses.

A booklet entitled "Scholarships, Fellowships, Educational Grants and Loans for R.N.'s" is available for 75¢ from the National League for Nursing, 10 Columbus Circle, New York, New York, 10019.

At one time the reason many students trained for nursing was strictly financial. Today, the high cost of training and higher blue collar wages have decreased the economic advantage significantly. The reason that you are in nursing training today should be because you desire more than anything else to be a nurse. Nursing can help you to realize your potential. Your education will cost you time and money. If you are willing to make the necessary sacrifice, you can succeed.

NOTES

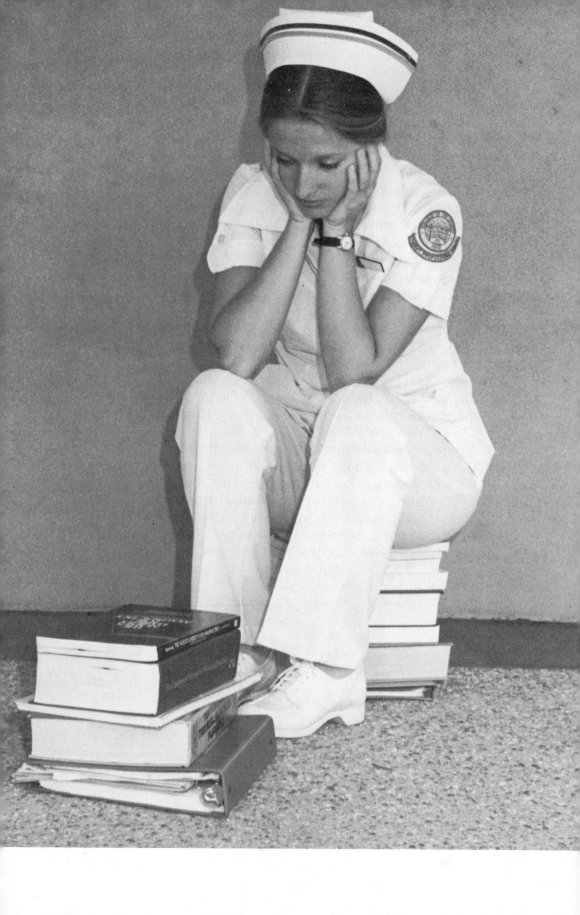

Chapter 9

Adjustment to Nursing Education

Nursing education will offer you many new opportunities. You will meet interesting people with a variety of ideas and values. You will hear new points of view from teachers and new friends. You will have the opportunity to make decisions. Intellectual challenges not present in high school or in jobs are before you.

There will be a great deal of hustle and bustle at school and at the hospital. There is always something happening. You can go in many different directions or you can stay put. You don't have to get involved in everything right away. Take the time to find out about the groups you are interested in. After making decisions, don't wait to be invited; express your interest. You can gain a great deal from extracurricular activities. They go a long way in the development of interpersonal skills.

Don't limit yourself to one group of friends who think as you do. You have an opportunity to form lasting friendships with people having diverse viewpoints. Both formal and informal groups can be very meaningful. They also help to fulfill your human needs of recognition and belonging.

For leadership or administrative positions future prospective employers will be interested in the groups you belonged to at college. If you didn't belong to any groups, they could possibly assume that you had an adjustment problem, or they might consider you dull. Holding office in a club or organization will be regarded as an indication of leadership ability.

Sororities, fraternities, and other social clubs have lost much of their former importance on campus. These groups, however, can be particularly helpful to students who have difficulty relating to others. If you tend to be a shy or retiring person, extracurricular clubs and groups can help you to be more outgoing. You need not join every social group on campus. Start by choosing one or two that seem to share your values or interests. A small effort on your part can bring large returns in the form of new friends and new interpersonal skills. An ability to deal with people in an efficient and humane way is vital for nurses. Social clubs can be your practice arena for development of "people skills."

Some students adopt "far out" ideas to get attention. As members of an unusual group, they feel that they achieve status and recognition. Often this type of group attracts loners or those who normally have trouble relating to their peers. As mentioned above, if you are this type of person, we feel that the more traditional social groups and organizations can help you to overcome your shyness. Membership in a bizarre group or cult may actually separate you still further from campus life and nursing care.

Often such cults are religious in nature. Overly shy people may be attracted to them because they offer a sense of belonging. It is natural to want to feel that you're part of a group rather than an outsider; but beware of groups whose members are fanatical in their allegiance or which require that you give up your individuality. You are at a point in your life where you're just beginning to pursue your personal goals. Up till now you may have been in school because you had to be. Much of your life may have been regulated by your parents and teachers. As a nursing student you have the chance to make your own decisions. Why give up the privilege of personal choice by joining a group that requires you to place their goals ahead of your own?

True religion can help you. It can give you courage and strengthen your relationship with God. Don't be ashamed of being a religious person. But before you get involved with any group, be sure you understand the group fully and what your involvement will entail. Remember that the peer group or groups with which you become involved at school are going to play a major part in your happiness and effectiveness as a nursing student.

This may be the first time you have shared a room with someone other than a family member. If you have the opportunity to choose a roommate, look for someone with the same values, but not necessarily the same interests. Shared values mean that you'll be compatible; divergent interests mean that your roommate may introduce you to new ideas and activities that will help you to grow.

ROOM-MATES

To live in harmony with someone else requires some adjustment in your life style. The all-important art of getting along with people — whether they are roommates, lovers, spouse, or patients — requires a great deal of give and take. You must learn to respect your roommate and yourself.

The following simple rules of living will help you get along with your roommate as well as with others. They apply to college and to life in general.

Respect the privacy of your roommate. Don't pry into personal affairs. If your roommate wants you to know, he or she will tell you.

Respect also your roommate's social privacy. Just as you have friends, so does your roommate. Don't become an uninvited tagalong.

Don't borrow your roommate's possessions or use his or her toiletries without permission. Often it is these little annoyances that are the most irritating.

Treat your roommate as an equal. At home you may have ordered younger brothers and sisters around, but don't try to give orders to your roommate.

Respond in a positive way to the achievements and possessions of your roommate. Some people try to build themselves up by belittling others.

When you do have an argument, try to be fair and to treat your roommate with respect. Remember that there are always at least two sides to an argument.

Try to foster a considerate, nonthreatening social interaction. Avoid competing for the same dates or positions whenever alternatives are available.

Be modest about your possessions and those of your family.

If you discuss your roommate with other people, be fair. Try to say only the kinds of things you would want your roommate to say about you.

If it is necessary for you to be critical of an action of your roomate, learn to criticize in a positive way. You must allow people to keep their self-respect.

Show that you are interested in your roommate as a person. Learn to listen to your roommate. Many people tend to hear what they want to hear, rather than what is being said. If you are having problems with your roommate, wait until you are both calm before discussing them. Avoid trying to solve problems when either of you is in an emotional state.

While your roommate isn't going to be perfect, neither are you. Your roommate is a human being with feelings that you should respect.

PATIENTS   The patients you deal with are individuals with human feelings. It can be difficult to deal with people having serious problems. It requires emotional stability on your part.

Some nurses seem to treat patients coldly, as objects rather than as human beings. This appearance of not caring is generally a defense mechanism that the person has created to avoid emotional involvement. Putting the patient at an emotional arm's length is an inappropriate protective measure. Other nurses rush about with a busy-busy attitude. This also is a protective measure to avoid dealing with emotions. They find that if they hurry from task to task, they don't have to think. If you find it difficult to be warm and responsive to patients, try to uncover the root of your problem. Perhaps you're afraid that if you allow yourself to care about your patients then their discomfort will be too painful for you. Perhaps you fear rejection. There are many reasons for putting a wall around oneself, but as a nurse you are committed to giving and sharing of yourself with others. Your patients need your respect and your personal involvement as much as they need your professional and technical skills.

The first step toward developing a giving attitude is to assess yourself honestly. Talk to nurses and to fellow students. You may be surprised to find that they share many of your anxieties and fears. Your school counselor can provide sound and sympathetic advice.

One of the best ways to deal with your emotions is by open discussion in post-clinical conferences. You will find that you are not unique in your feelings. Everyone in the health care field experiences guilt and the feeling that they could have or should have done more for a patient. Such worries are normal. Don't keep your problems inside. Others have feelings, insecurities, and doubts also. Use of your nursing group for support will help keep everything in a realistic perspective.

Shoptalk in private helps to relieve tension. Some of the jokes you hear may be somewhat morbid, but they serve the purpose of relieving tension. Great care should be taken that this type of discussion takes place beyond the hearing of people who are not professionally involved.

Most patient dissatisfaction with nursing care is based not so much on actual deficiencies in the care received as on imagined inadequacies. The problem is primarily one of nurse-patient communication.

COMMUNI-CATION WITH PATIENTS

The patient must be made to realize that he or she is important to you and that you are interested. Address patients by name rather than as "Dearie" or "Honey." It is hard for many patients who are unable to care for themselves to maintain dignity. You must do all you can to maintain your patient's sense of self-esteem.

We communicate in many ways. Besides the spoken word, facial expressions, posture, dress, inflections in the voice, gestures, touch, and even what we don't say carry messages. If you do not understand the patient, you cannot possibly give complete care. The communication skills you will learn in your nursing training will aid you in every aspect of your life.

Make sure that the patient fully understands what you are trying to convey. A patient's own past experiences and feelings will affect the way information is received. Take into consideration such factors as the patient's level of education and familiarity with the hospital environment. Many patients are afraid of hospitals and are intimidated by the highly technical language that is being used all around them. Avoid using technical terminology, especially with patients from poor or underprivileged backgrounds. On the other hand, don't be condescending or evasive with patients. Their trust in you will be decreased if they feel that you are holding back or disguising the truth.

Your words, actions, dress, and posture must communicate to the patient that you are a trained professional but that you also care. A positive and efficient approach shows professionalism and relieves the patient's anxiety.

Nurse-patient communication is a two-way street. You must learn to listen closely to the patient and to ask questions. Often patients are reluctant to talk about what is really on their minds. A patient who fears that she has breast cancer may talk about a friend or relative who had cancer. Be alert for these clues by paying attention to the patient's tone of voice and gestures and other nonverbal messages.

STRESSES OF NURSE TRAINING

If you are overly shy and also have serious problems in relating to others, you should seek help. Your counselor will be able to help you find psychological treatment.

At some time or another you are going to feel lonely. It is a normal feeling; everyone experiences it at some time. You can have this feeling even in the midst of a crowd. One common cure for loneliness is to get involved in some outside activity. Loneliness occurs when you feel separated from the world around you. By participating in some group activity you may be able to re-establish your sense of belonging. Unfortunately, loneliness tends to make us withdraw further and further into our own private sorrows, which in turn intensifies the feeling of loneliness. If you can reach out just a little, you're on your way back to happiness. At first you may have to push yourself to do things and join in, but for each effort that you make you'll find your emotional balance is restored a little more. Participation in group sports or heavy physical activity is a good way to be with people and to release nervous energy at the same time.

Nurse training has built-in stresses. To start with you will be thrown into crisis situations. You will be exposed to people who are undergoing physical and emotional traumas. Couple this with competition for grades and long class and clinical hours and it becomes very clear that this is a point in your life when you are likely to be highly emotional.

Severe depression may be caused by a wide variety of events — poor grades, things not working out as planned, health worries, financial problems, a broken romance, sexual problems, loneliness, arguments, parental pressures, feelings of inadequacy, worry over the state of the world, a clinical experience, and even fear of things that just might happen but probably won't. Often the problem can be cumulative, the result of many small incidents. You may find yourself feeling depressed without really being sure of the reason. One of the best ways to free yourself from depression is to talk to a counselor or friend. By bringing your worries into the open you'll be better equipped to deal with them. Many of your fears may be lessened or eliminated just by talking about them and seeing that they're not as serious as they seem. Other worries become less burdensome when you face up to them and develop a strategy for dealing with them. Don't be ashamed to seek help. As the first step in overcoming depression, seeking help is a strong sign of health on your part.

SUICIDE

Suicide is the second leading cause of student deaths (accidents are first). Suicide sometimes seems a very simple solution to a difficult or stressful situation. There may even be a desire to "get even." A depressed person may say to himself or herself, "They'll be sorry they treated me that way," or "I'll show them." Suicide thus is thought of as a weapon against others, but, of course, such deaths are tragedies, and the suffering they cause profits no one.

Most suicides are not successful, largely because people who contemplate suicide don't really want to die. What they really want is for someone to care about them, to know of their unhappiness. This is evidenced by the fact that many suicides call friends or relatives to tell them that they are going to kill themselves. Such an action should be regarded as a cry for help.

Anxieties, coupled with lack of sleep, are mental danger signals. If a student talks about death or suicide while under pressure, someone should remain with the student. A usually active person who starts to stay in bed for long periods or to just sit and stare into space may be emotionally upset. If you are seriously worried about your mental state, or that of a friend, you should seek professional aid. Avoid self-help type encounter groups that are not under expert direction. These sessions, in which everyone says what he or she really thinks, can be extremely ego damaging if not run properly.

Men have been taught since childhood that showing emotions is for girls and is not manly. They "keep a stiff upper lip" and bottle things within themselves. This attitude frequently leads to serious emotional problems. Though some feel that the women's liberation movement is a mixed blessing, it at least has helped us to outgrow these restrictive ideas about how men should act.

"SECOND TERM TRAP"

Often after a successful first term, everything seems to go wrong. These problems are caused by a number of factors. Upon getting good grades the first term many students ease off a little, which often is too much. The over-confidence of a "this isn't so bad" attitude can result in disastrous grades. Also, by the second term the student is starting to get involved in outside activities, which can result in neglect of education. To some students, their extracurricular activities become more important than their education. You should be aware of this "trap."

LOVE AND SEX

At this stage in your life, many of your problems will be sex-related. Sexual feelings are natural. Not so many years ago most people wouldn't discuss sexual matters even with their own spouses. Today, people are more apt to talk about sex openly.

We, as human beings, are naturally gregarious. That is, we like other people. We want to feel wanted by others. We need recognition by others. We have the desire to make strong friendships. "Meaningful relationship" is a term frequently used for this type of attachment.

Dating during college should not be a game of chess, with each party looking for an advantage. It should be mutually beneficial and enjoyable. A healthy attitude can build both egos. Dating should be a comfortable relationship, not a win-lose competition.

Don't build relationships into something they are not. Let them develop on their own. Unrealistic expectations can lead to severe letdowns. Many students are in love with love. They want to be in love so much that they convince themselves they are in love. Sex should not be confused with love. Love is an emotion, and although words cannot adequately describe emotions, it can be said that when you love someone your center of interest transfers from yourself to another, who replaces you as being number one in your thoughts and future.

In college many students seek casual sexual relationships. They feel that if both parties are mature, they can have a convenient relationship without becoming emotionally involved. However, you should realize that the desire not to become emotionally involved doesn't mean that you won't. A relationship can seldom be ended without some emotional scars.

At present there is a tendency toward more open, nonconforming sexual relationships (such as bisexuality or homosexuality) at college. Some of these relationships are not just open but are practically advertised, whereas in the past they would have been kept highly secret. You should consider the effect of such relationships on your family and upon your partner's family. Even if such unconventional relationships are more socially acceptable than in the past, thoughtlessness is not. Your desire to be open should be tempered by consideration for others who may be unable to cope with your beliefs. People who depart from the norm in their behavior face many difficulties. Tact and delicacy are extremely important.

Largely because of lack of understanding, many people have sexual hangups. They have mixed feelings, fantasies, and fears that they feel are abnormal. Such fantasies and thoughts, although they may be frightening to you, may be perfectly normal. Sexual problems should be talked out with a counselor.

VENEREAL DISEASE

Venereal disease has increased at an alarming rate. Some of the new varieties of disease are resistant to penicillin and are not easily cured. The two basic types of venereal disease are syphilis and gonorrhea. In syphilis, the first symptom is a sore or chancre (which often is not detected in women). Because the symptom disappears does not mean you are well, since syphilis does not go away unless treated. If left untreated, syphilis can lead to brain damage, insanity, damage to other organs, paralysis, and death. Gonorrhea, also known as "clap," normally has an initial symptom of burning during urination, although 80 percent of women with gonorrhea have no symptoms. Gonorrhea, if untreated, can result in sterility, as well as heart and brain damage. Gonorrhea during pregnancy can cause blindness in the newborn.

Should you have any symptoms of venereal disease,

you have a duty to notify your partner at once. The only sure way to know whether or not you are infected is a physical examination. If you want more information, check with your college medical office or your own physician.

Unwanted pregnancies still occur despite the ready availability of contraceptives, primarily because sex isn't always planned, and contraceptives are not always absolute protection. Generally, marriages entered into primarily because of pregnancy have two strikes against them. Considering the fact that approximately half of all marriages end in divorce, the chances of a forced marriage succeeding are not very good.

Often students marry for marriage's sake. Everyone else is getting married, and the students decide it isn't such a bad idea. Marriage for this reason or to escape parental control or some other problem generally means real trouble later on. Marriage is one of the most serious steps you can take. The responsibilities — and rewards — are great. Make this all-important decision carefully and it will bring you great happiness. A hasty or impulsive decision can cause much regret.

Many students are still in the process of growing up, still changing and developing their personalities rapidly. You and your partner should be very sure that you know yourselves and each other well enough to make this lifelong commitment.

DRUGS

Drug problems exist in nursing school just as they do elsewhere. Nurses (like doctors) can be prone to take drugs. Self-medication is common because it is available. For basic drug information, see the Appendix. For drug problems, your counselor can direct you to professional help.

GETTING ALONG WITH YOUR PARENTS AND FAMILY

At one time you knew that your parents could protect you and solve all your problems. You regarded them as very special people. As you matured, you discovered that your parents are not any different from other people. They have the same problems and feelings as everyone else. When an image is shattered, people tend to go to the other extreme. Upon seeing their parents' imperfections for the first time, adolescents may feel that their parents have no good qualities at all. You might feel that they interfere with your life. When your parents force something on you or tell you that you cannot do something, you might very well do the opposite if you have the chance. This is not so much a rejection of the ideas of your parents; it is more an act of rebellion. It applies to sex, drinking, and many other actions.

The fact that your parents still look upon you as a child when you want to be regarded as an equal often precipitates conflict. Parental conflict also results because you may be dependent on your parents for most of your needs, but you resent this dependency. Your parents might feel that as long as they are paying the bills, you should do what they say.

Understanding your parents is a two-way street. Your parents are under stress, just as you are. Getting along under stress can be difficult. Your parents may have financial stress or a fear of failing. If you fail, they may feel they have failed. They worry about what can happen to you. Some parents, although financially successful, regard themselves as failures for one reason or another. They might fear that you will end up like them. They might desire to live vicariously through you and want you to have and do the things they did not have or do.

Your parents received no special training in how to be parents. Many times they did not know whether to be tough or lenient, and they may have been inconsistent in their treatment of you. Their feelings toward you may have resulted in family conflict. They are afraid of doing the wrong thing but are unsure of what is right.

You should regard your parents as beautiful people. They have feelings. Their egos need building up just as yours does. Give some words of encouragement. Make them feel successful. Allow for their mistakes. Even if you know they are mistaken, remember that they are trying to help you.

SPOUSES

Your husband or wife probably has no idea of the difficulty of your educational preparation. Your program is very demanding, and this can lead to marital stress. You must be careful that you do not neglect your family. Plan for family time and activities. Take a few minutes each day to tell your spouse about your day and its problems. This communication is essential. It will help your spouse understand your situation, and the simple process of verbalizing problems will help to relieve your own stress.

Married students may feel that when they are with their family that they should be studying and when studying they may feel they should be with their family. They may fear poor grades because they feel they must reward their family with good grades because they are sacrificing so much. Married students should realize that these guilt feelings are normal. However, feelings of guilt must not be allowed to consume your energy and adversely affect your education or your family life.

You should be aware that pregnancy of a student or spouse can become an added burden. It can create a crisis situation as to nursing education as well as to family life.

Even though you may feel great stress you should consciously try to be a happy person with your family. Your nursing preparation should not be at the expense of your family.

Make the most of the time spent in nursing. It can make you into a more sensitive and understanding human being as well as provide new horizons of knowledge. Your experiences can go a long way toward making the rest of your life more rewarding.

NOTES

NOTES

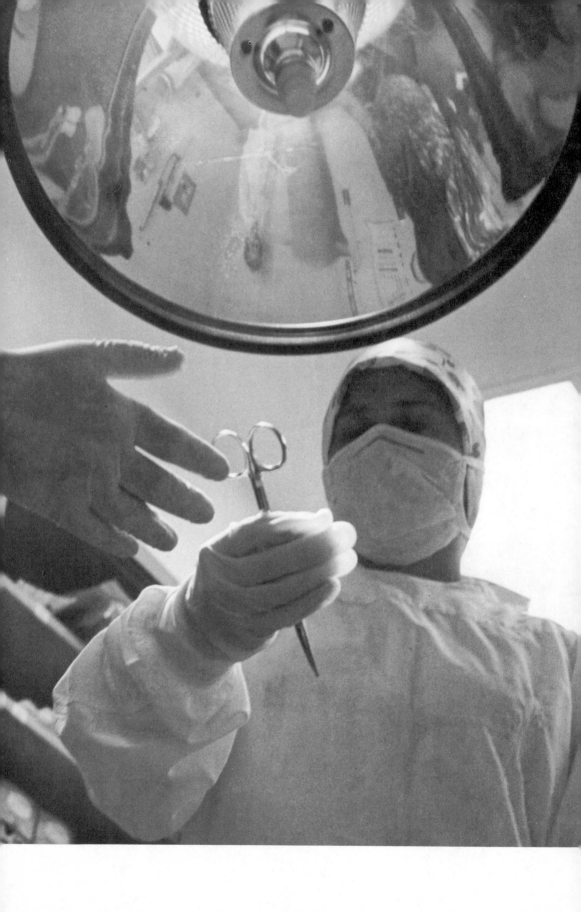

Chapter 10

Employment During and After College

As a result of the current economic situation and the increasing realization that marriage is made up of two equal partners, women (both single and married) are becoming accepted as a natural and permanent part of our work force.

You are fortunate in having chosen a career field that will give you great personal satisfaction as well as employment opportunities wherever you may be.

Work experience within the health care field prior to receiving your degree will give you a great deal of leverage in finding permanent career employment, especially if there are limited job openings in a particular area of nursing that interests you. In addition, such experience often allows you to negotiate a higher starting salary than someone with no work background would expect. As an example, assume your career goal is to work with emotionally disturbed children. Summer work in a clinic or summer camp dealing with these children would be very valuable in terms of your career as well as being personally rewarding.

Direct job experience during college offers several other advantages. It gives you valuable insight into curriculum planning. You might see the need to take courses other than those originally planned or even to modify or change the emphasis of your career program. It can also reveal whether or not you have been correct in your career choice. Naturally, if you are going to change any of your career goals, the sooner in your educational program that you do so, the easier it will be.

Many students who obtain summer employment at hospitals and prove themselves dedicated employees end up being offered full-time jobs. At one university that has a program for providing jobs directly related to the student's career field, over 50 percent of the students receive full-time job offers from these summer jobs.

Whether or not you work during your nursing preparation, you are going to have to obtain employment in the future. All too often, highly trained students feel that they are lost after graduation. They feel they are being set loose in a sink-or-swim situation, with no counselors or instructors to give them guidance.

Just as it is possible to plan an education to fulfill your individual needs, you can plan to obtain employment based on those same needs. If you wish to supplement your education with directly related work experience during college, your job search should really begin shortly after you start college. If you have a career goal, or even areas that interest you, then you are ready for the first step, which is to analyze the market.

ASSESSING THE MARKET

First you should consider what employment opportunities are available in the area. The purpose of this preliminary search for job sites is to find summer employment, and possibly even part-time employment during the school year, within a field that interests you.

Of course, the primary market for nurses is at hospitals. But consider this: Nurses are employed by federal, state, county, and city governments, industrial firms, nursing homes, private duty nurse services, passenger ships, camps, schools, commercial business, medical offices, and even private individuals. Don't overlook the student employment office on campus. They might have a job that fits right in with your career plan. In addition, your instructors can probably supply you with employment suggestions within your area of interest.

After your initial research, you should list all the jobs that you are interested in. For health care facilities within your geographical area, you will want to present yourself in person for an interview. For firms outside the area, you will usually have to rely on letters or telephone calls, because of the time and cost of traveling. Before you personally contact a local employer, you should obtain as much information about the employer as possible. Among sources of information are friends who might know an employee and members of your nursing faculty.

Your next step is to obtain an interview with potential employers. There is a strategy to this important telephone call; a carefully worded request can help to ensure the reply you want. Consider the following example:

THE INITIAL INTERVIEW: SUMMER AND PART-TIME JOBS

"Mr. Thomas, my name is Frances Brown, and I'm a first year nursing student at State College. I plan to specialize in psychiatric nursing. I'd like to stop by and talk to you for just a few minutes. Would Friday at two o'clock be convenient for you?"

You are not telling Mr. Thomas what you want, only that you are a student in a field in which he is very interested. Most people enjoy talking to students about their work. By setting a time you make it very easy for Mr. Thomas to say yes. If Mr. Thomas can't make it at two o'clock, he will probably suggest another time when it will be convenient for you to stop by. Don't try to schedule an appointment for Monday morning, since this is usually one of the busiest times.

When you go to an interview, keep in mind that the people doing the interviewing are generally older and more conservative than you are. You should, therefore, dress in a way that you feel the person interviewing you would expect of the model nursing student. Most important is that you look clean and neat. Don't chew gum or smoke. Avoid heavy perfume, scented deodorant, or aftershave lotion. Use of a breath freshener is a good idea. Walk erect, and greet the person you wish to see with a firm handshake. Make sure that you pronounce the interviewer's name correctly.

At this point, Mr. Thomas does not know that you want to work for him. Approach the subject by explaining your career goals. Tell him about your courses and your curricular plans, tailoring your description to his field. Rehearse what you're going to say before the actual interview.

Ask a friend to listen to your speech and to point out any inconsistency or repetition. A lengthy autobiographical explanation of your goals, plans, and ideas is not necessary. Be brief and concise. Include only those aspects of your plans that are directly relevant to the interviewer's work.

After describing your situation, explain that you are interested in what the employer is doing, and why, and that you would like to have work experience there for the summer (or part-time and summer, if applicable). You are really saying, "I know what you are doing, I am interested in it, and I would like to play a part in your work."

This approach will probably be well received. Keep in mind that you are talking to a person about a position that may not even exist. If you have sold yourself, there is a good possibility that a job will be created for you. This is especially true of summer jobs, when vacations result in many scheduling problems. Actually, if you are hired because of vacation problems, the chances are you will be exposed to a variety of work situations, which will greatly enhance the value of your experience.

If the interviewer seems interested but does not actually offer you a position, ask for a job. As an example, you might say: "I believe that I've shown you that I'm an energetic and dedicated student. Would you like me to work for you this summer? By a few words, you have made it easy for the employer to make an immediate decision.

Generally, *personnel offices* should be avoided for summer jobs. Unless there is actually an opening, your response will be a polite letter stating that they are not hiring. The personnel office is not likely to create a summer position; your chances are much better with a working level supervisor.

Don't feel that you've wasted the interview if you are not offered a job. Contacts are an important part of career development. Although your interviewer does not have a job for you at this point, she or he is still a valuable resource. He or she has a position of some importance in a field that you wish to learn more about, and you can probably obtain additional career guidance from him or her. People are generally flattered when you ask them for guidance, and they usually will try to help you. Ask for suggestions about elective courses. Find out about further nursing specialization and future employment prospects. Ask your interviewer whether he or she can suggest any other employer who could use someone with your nursing interests for summer employment. If a suggestion is made, find out who specifically to contact. You will then be able to say, "Mr. Thomas of St. Luke's Hospital suggested that I speak to you." This personal approach generally has a positive effect.

　　Never leave an unsuccessful job interview without giving a résumé to the employer. An example of a simple résumé appropriate for summer or part-time work is shown in the box. Whenever possible, limit your résumé to one page. Employers do not have time to sift through several pages in order to determine your value as an employee, especially if you're seeking only summer or part-time work. Brevity and conciseness are as important here as at the interview itself.

Résumé:　Frances Brown
1476 Maple Lane
College City, MO 52816
(726) 589–4168

Objective:　Summer employment as a nurse aide in a health care facility specializing in psychiatric care and treatment. This will serve to reinforce my career goal as a nurse specializing in psychiatric work.

Education:　Currently completing my freshman year at State College, enrolled in their nursing program.

At Center City High School I graduated 12th in my class of 189 students.

Previous Employment:　Part-time employment at Foundation for Retarded Citizens past two years.

Organizations and Awards:　Scout Leader, Vice-President of Student Council in high school. Winner of Hiram Chambers Scholarship Award.

Personal Data:　Age 19
　　　　　　　　　Height:　5' 5"; Weight:　115 lb.
　　　　　　　　　Health:　Excellent

References supplied upon request.

The *Objective* sets forth your goals in a clear fashion. It also gives you an opportunity to sell yourself. The self-assessment exercises from Chapter 2 helped you to develop your goals into a well-organized plan for the future. Your notes from that chapter should be useful in writing a brief Objectives paragraph for your résumé.

The *Education* section should show directly related experience. If you ranked high in your high school graduating class, this should be indicated.

The purpose of listing *Previous Employment* is to show that you are familiar with the working world. If you have had specifically related job experience, this should, of course, be emphasized. If you have had no job history, omit this section completely.

Organizations and Awards will show your prospective employer that you are a well-rounded person with many interests. If you have had any position of leadership, you should include it, as it will indicate to a prospective employer that you have executive ability. Employers normally react favorably to religious work, such as teaching Sunday school. A religious person is generally viewed as mature and stable.

The *Personal Data* section is not necessary. Its purpose is to show that you are in good health and are physically able to do the work required. It also gives the reader of the résumé a clearer image of who you are. However, this optional paragraph can have a negative effect. For example, if you're overweight or underweight, or if an employer might consider you too young or too old for the work you seek, your safest course is to leave out the personal data section. Once you actually obtain an interview, you can present your case in person and show the interviewer that these factors will not interfere with your job responsibilities.

References are required by many employers as part of a formal job application. They should not be submitted with résumés, nor should "To Whom It May Concern" letters of recommendation be attached. Employers know that your references are going to be positive, or you wouldn't list them.

Your résumé should contain no negative data. The purpose of the résumé is to give just enough information so that the reader will want to investigate you further. It's really like a short advertisement to get the buyer to inspect the product.

If you are interested in more than one career area, you'll probably need several different résumés, each aimed directly at a specific career. Keep in mind that employers look at résumés in terms of specific job prospects. Your information should be as directly relevant to a particular position as possible.

SALARY NEGOTIA-TION

During your interview you should not ask questions about salary or fringe benefits. It might be naive on the part of employers, but they expect employees to be primarily interested in the work and not in the benefits. The proper time to discuss wages is after you are offered a job.

If the employer asks you what you want in the line of salary, it is best to state that you would expect to be treated in a fair manner but that the job is of primary importance. If you name a salary that the interviewer considers too high, he or she probably will not offer you a job. If you state a salary that seems too low, he or she might wonder why you're willing to work for such small wages. In many hospitals and institutions wages are set without room for negotiation.

Keep in mind that in the long run, work experience directly related to your career area is worth far more than nonrelated work experience, regardless of salary.

CORRE-SPONDENCE

For summer jobs outside your geographical area, you will have to rely on the mails.

If one of your nursing instructors is willing to recommend you to an employer he or she knows, this can be extremely effective. By stating in your letter, "Professor Alva Hodgekins of the Nursing School at State College suggested I write to you," you have opened the door (providing, of course, that the recipient holds Professor Hodgekins in high esteem).

Never address a letter to Personnel Director, Supervisor, or just the firm or institution name. This is much like your receiving a letter addressed to "Occupant." Find out the name of the person who would be directly responsible for hiring you. Perhaps someone on campus — the placement office, an instructor, of even a classmate — has this information. If not, a brief note (or phone call, if you can afford it) to the personnel department, asking the name of the supervisor in your area of interest, should provide you with the information you need.

While you wish to avoid personnel people at this stage of the job search, you do not want to alienate them. Therefore, a copy of your covering letter and résumé should be sent to the personnel department.

It is far more difficult to sell yourself on paper to a person who perhaps does not have a formal job opening than it is in person. Therefore, your letter and résumé must be carefully worded. One example of a letter of introduction is shown in the box.

Donaldson Engineering
4725 Midway Boulevard
Adonburg, Ohio 58731

Attention: Mr Henry Johnson, Director of Plant Services

Dear Mr. Johnson:

I am extremely interested in your innovative Industrial Health Facility as set forth in the article in the December issue of *Health Monthly*.

I am a freshman in the School of Nursing at State University and am very interested in obtaining a position for the summer with your firm. As you will see from my enclosed résumé, my educational goals and experience to date are directly related to Industrial Health Care.

I will call you Thursday, March 2, to see when it might be convenient to meet with you personally.

Yours truly,

This letter immediately shows Mr. Johnson that you know something about the firm and are interested in a particular summer job. By letting him know that you will call him, Mr. Johnson is forced to think about whether or not he can use you. If, when you call, you are able to get an interview, chances are they are seriously considering hiring you. Generally, a firm will not ask someone to travel any distance for an interview, especially for only a summer position, unless they expect to be hiring.

Of course, if you are unable to get an interview when you call, all it has cost you is a phone call. (Never call collect when inquiring for a job, as this is both rude and extremely poor strategy.)

If you cannot afford to travel a great distance for a summer job interview, and if even long-distance phone calls will seriously impair your budget, then a simple closing sentence, such as the following, is appropriate: "I am looking forward to hearing from you."

Before you graduate, recruiters from various hospitals and institutions will probably be coming to your campus. Generally, either the guidance or student employment office will post notices of these interviews. If you are interested in any of the employers, you should sign up for an interview. Before the interview, learn all you can about the employer. Recruiters complain that most college students coming to interviews don't have the slightest idea of what the firm or institution they are being interviewed by really does. By proper research, you can increase your competitive chances considerably.

COLLEGE RECRUITING

Since these college interviewers often ask you to fill out a formal employment application, be sure to have your social security number, names and addresses of former employers and supervisors, and names and addresses of at least three references. References should be written by people to whom your interviewer can relate, such as people in the same general field or professors in your major field of study.

Sometimes college recruiters have the power to hire on the spot. More often, if they are interested, they will pay your expenses for a trip to their facility, so that you will have a first-hand opportunity to see what they do. The visit will give the employer a chance to learn about you, and you will have the opportunity to learn about the employer.

You may have a series of interviews at a single institution. The personnel department will be interested in your personal adjustment and the prospects of your continued career growth. The people you would be working for (or with) are interested in what kind of a fellow worker you would be and what you really know from your education and past experience.

These interviews are a two-way street. You must convince the employer that you are the right person for the position, and the employer must convince you that the job is the right job for you. Both employer and prospective employee must be satisfied.

Besides waiting for recruiters to come to your school, there is a great deal that you can be doing during your last year for your career job search.

Since employers cannot visit every school, often they simply send letters to the schools (especially the smaller colleges) stating their employment needs. Your school's employment office will have this information as well as applications for some of the jobs. If the employer is interested, he will contact you.

If there are other schools in your area, find out which employers are visiting them. Generally, there will be no problem in utilizing their services.

If you receive a job offer and are not sure about whether or not you should accept, ask for some time to consider it. Employers recognize that this is a major decision for you and will allow you time to weigh all factors. After all, careful consideration on your part is to the employer's benefit as well, because if you choose your job situation wisely you'll be a more productive and valuable worker.

Because of shortages in nursing, you can expect several offers. All too often graduates accept the first job offer they receive or else the one that offers the most money, without really analyzing whether the job is one they will be happy with. While no job is going to be ideal in every aspect, and some readjustment of priorities may be necessary, the job you accept must fulfill your basic employment needs.

Professional publications list many positions, as does the *Wall Street Journal*. Your school library probably has newspapers from other areas. You can also check newsstands for out-of-town papers or order the Sunday edition, with the large want-ad section, directly from the publisher.

Nurse registries have information on positions available within a community. You can locate these registries through your telephone yellow pages.

You should also consider placing an ad in a professional journal dealing with your career area. This is especially helpful if you are looking for a highly specialized position.

Other people can help you to find a position. Check with your instructors, current and past; they generally have many students already employed at various levels within health care facilities in your area. If they can help, they will.

You should consider taking the Professional and Administrative Career Examination (PACE) during your senior year. This is the entry level examination for federal employment and gets you on the Civil Service Register. Uncle Sam is our largest employer and has positions in every imaginable discipline. When you get on the Civil Service Register, you should send Standard Form 171 (employment application) to each government agency that you feel could use your training. Besides sending the forms to the agency in Washington, D.C., you can also send them to each of their regional offices.

The Veterans Administration uses direct applications rather than the regular Civil Service Examinations. These applications are available at any VA facility.

Some private employment services are very worthwhile, especially those specializing in a particular career area. They usually charge fees equal to one month's earnings. Often the employer will pay part or all of this fee. You should read carefully any contract you sign, as some firms have clauses making them your exclusive representative and obligating you to a fee no matter how you obtain a position.

Avoid advance-fee career consultants. Generally, these firms offer very little for a large fee. State employment agencies are usually worthless for college graduates. Generally, people contacting them are looking for cheap labor.

Contacting executive recruiters is also a waste of time. These recruiters have a few specific jobs to be filled and are looking for people with a great deal of experience for these positions. They do not look for jobs to fit people. Because of this, it would be sheer luck for your qualifications to come across a recruiter's desk at the same time that there was an opening requiring your qualifications.

Avoid having your résumé prepared by résumé shops. "Canned" résumés usually are so general that they are discarded. You should prepare your own personal résumé, tailored to specific jobs. This may mean a change in emphasis on a résumé for various positions.

Writing letters and résumés and making phone calls will keep you busy. Finding the right job isn't always easy, and the more specialized the job, generally the longer it is going to take you. Use the basic techniques described in this chapter for writing résumés and letters.

For experience, show only applicable work experience. If this is lacking, then list courses you have taken that are directly related to the job you are seeking.

For your job interviews, you should be prepared for the following:

1. A question that allows you to tell about yourself. Be organized and give data that fits in with the needs of the position being applied for.

2. A question about why you wish to work for the firm, hospital, or institution. You should be able to show how your goals coincide with the firm's goals.

3. A question about your future aspirations. Your future goals should be progressive, along the same line as the position you are applying for. If not, you are probably applying for the wrong position.

4. A chance to ask questions. This gives you an excellent opportunity to show the depth of your knowledge concerning the employer.

5. Questions about social adjustment. Professional interviewers will ask questions designed to determine whether or not you have any social problems and to reveal the type of person you are in terms of your attitudes and values.

For further information about writing résumés and letters, as well as specific questions that you can expect in an interview, I recommend my *Work Experience Handbook*, published by Canfield Press.

Over one million jobs are filled each month in the United States. It is not enough to just find a job. You must strive for a position that meets your own individual needs.

NOTES

Appendix A

Your College Information

Fill in the following checklist for a ready reference of important information about your school and community services.

Activities card (where to obtain): _____

_____

_____

Advisor
    My faculty advisor is: _____
    Office location: _____ Phone: _____
    Office hours are: _____

Alcohol (campus rules regarding alcoholic beverages): _____

_____

_____

Athletics
    For information on intramural athletics: _____

_____

_____

    For information on intercollegiate athletics: _____

_____

_____

Attendance (rules about being dropped): _____

_____

_____

_____

Audiovisual center (location): _____

_____

_____

Banking
    Location: _____
    Hours: _____

Behavioral problems (information on suspension and expulsion): _____

_____

_____

_____

_____

_____

Birth control information available at: _____

_____

_____

_____

_____ Phone: _____

Book store
    Location: _____

_____

    Hours: _____

Bulletin boards (posting information): _____

_____

_____

Bursar's office (location): _____

_____ Phone: _____

Carpool information: _____

_____

_____

Catalog (copies available at): _____

_____

_____

Check cashing
    Checks may be cashed at: _____

_____

_____

    Hours: _____

Child care center: _____

_____

_____

_____

Clubs and organizations

Name of Clubs	Person to Contact
_____	_____
_____	_____
_____	_____
_____	_____
_____	_____
_____	_____
_____	_____
_____	_____
_____	_____

_____

_____

Copy center:
    Location: _____
    Phone: _____
    Individual copier
    Location: _____
    Cost: _____

Counselor
    My counselor is: _____
    Office location: _____ Phone: _____

    (Note: your advisor is a regular teacher, but your counselor is
    a professional trained to help you on career, curriculum, and
    personal problems.)

Counseling
    Educational and career counseling available at: _____
_____
_____ Phone: _____
    Personal counseling available at: _____
_____ Phone: _____

Crisis
    For serious problems such as suicide prevention or drugs or alcohol
    problems, contact: _____
_____
_____
_____
_____

Dean of Instruction: _____
    Office: _____ Phone: _____

Dean of Students: _____
    Office: _____ Phone: _____

Drug counseling and information
    Location: _____
_____
_____ Phone: _____

Educational opportunity program
    Location: _____
_____
_____ Phone: _____

Employment service
    Campus employment office: _____
_____ Phone: _____
    Community employment office: _____
_____ Phone: _____

Equal opportunity
    For problems involving discrimination, contact: _____
_____
_____
_____

Field studies programs:
  Information about off-campus study programs available from _____
_____

Financial aid office
  Location: _____
_____ Phone: _____

Food service
  Location: _____
_____ Hours: _____

Grades (where and when sent): _____
_____
_____

Grade points
  The school is on a _____ point system. An A is considered _____
  points, a B _____ points, a C _____ points and a D _____ points.
  Grade point average is computed by: _____
_____
_____
_____
_____

Graduate school information (where available): _____
_____
_____
_____
_____

Handicapped services: _____
_____
_____
_____

Health services:
    Student health office is located at: _____
_____ Phone: _____
    Hours: _____
    Additional information: _____
_____

Housing office
    Information for on-campus housing
        Location: _____ Phone: _____
    Information for off-campus housing
        Location: _____
_____ Phone: _____

Instructors' office hours

Name of Instructor	Office Location	Office Hours

Insurance information (student malpractice, health, life, and accident): ____
_____
_____
_____
_____
_____
_____

Laundry facilities
    Location: _____
_____
    Hours: _____

Legal aid
   Location: _____
_____
      Hours: _____
      Phone for appointment: _____

Library
   Campus location: _____
_____
      Hours: _____
      Late book charges: _____
_____
   Community location: _____
_____
      Hours: _____
      Late book charges: _____

   Hospital location: _____
   Medical society locations: _____

Lost and found office (location): _____
_____ Phone: _____

Mail: _____
_____

Maintenance office (location): _____
_____ Phone: _____

Maps
   Campus maps may be obtained at: _____
   Community maps may be obtained at: _____
_____

Mathematics laboratory: _____
_____
_____

Messages: _____
_____
_____

Newspaper: _____
_____

Notary public: _____
_____

Nursing associations: _____
_____

Parking information: _____
_____
_____
_____

Physical examination requirements: _____
_____

Police
  Campus location: _____
_____
_____

    Campus phone: _____
  Community location: _____
    Phone: _____

Press releases: _____
_____
_____
_____

Probation information and restrictions: _____
_____
_____
_____
_____

Reading laboratory: _____
_____
_____

Rooms (reservations for campus activities): _____

_____

_____

R.O.T.C. location: _____

_____ Phone: _____

Registration office: _____

_____ Phone: _____

Scholarship information: _____

_____

_____

_____

_____

Schedule of classes: _____

_____

_____

_____

_____

School activities
    Information will be available at: _____

_____

_____

_____

Smoking regulations: _____

_____

_____

Social Security benefit information: _____

_____

_____

Student government office: _____

_____

_____ Phone: _____

Telephones
   Use of campus phones: _____
_____

   Pay phones are located: _____
_____
_____

Television course information: _____
_____
_____
_____
_____
_____

Tickets
   Tickets for campus-held events will be available at: _____
_____
_____
_____

Transcripts (available at): _____
_____ Charge: _____

Tutorial program: _____
_____
_____
_____
_____

Typewriters (available for students): _____
_____ Hours: _____

Uniform requirements: _____
_____

Uniform suppliers: _____
_____

Veterans' office: _____
_____ Phone: _____

Welfare assistance information: _____
_____
_____
_____
_____

Withdrawal procedure: _____
_____
_____
_____

Work experience education: _____
_____
    Office location: _____
_____ Phone: _____

Women's center: _____
_____
_____
_____

Writing laboratory: _____
_____
_____
_____

Appendix B
Basic Drug Information

Alcohol.   It may seem strange to list alcohol as a drug, but drinking is a major college drug problem. Addiction to alcohol is a serious illness, for which the only cure is total abstinence.

Liquor is the social lubricant of our society. It makes people feel relaxed and generally uninhibited. Unlike the other drugs described in this section, drinking is an acceptable and even condoned social activity, and alcoholics can usually delude themselves and others about the seriousness of their addiction.

Alcoholism causes damage to the brain, liver, and blood vessels. If you think you are becoming a problem drinker, talk to your counselor; don't be afraid to seek help.

Amphetamines.   Because of their stimulant effect, these drugs are collectively known as ''speed.'' Among their effects, amphetamines stimulate the nervous system, depress appetite, and diminish fatigue (hence their popularity at exam time). As the effects of the drug wear off, the speed user experiences fatigue and depression.

Amphetamines have not been proved to be addictive, but their damaging effects to body and mind are beyond question. It is true that ''Speed kills.''

Barbiturates.   These drugs are usually prescribed for insomnia. Among the common brand names are Quaalude, Nembutal, and Seconal. In addition to making you sleepy, barbiturates can cause a feeling of euphoria, depression, and confusion or loss of memory. They are addictive, and withdrawal can be very difficult.

Cocaine.   Because of its cost, cocaine (or ''coke'') is generally considered a rich person's drug. You may have heard that cocaine is safe to use because it is not addictive. Bear in mind, however, that many drugs are psychologically addictive.

155

Unlike heroin, which slows down body processes, cocaine is a stimulant. The high that it provides is often followed by depression and a slowing of the heartbeat, which can be dangerous. Although it can be injected, cocaine usually is sniffed, and continual inhalation can damage the nasal passages.

Glue Sniffing. Inhaling the fumes of various flammables such as glue, gasoline, or nail polish is probably the most foolish and most dangerous of drug-related activities.

The fumes, which are usually sniffed from a plastic bag, produce intoxication. Sniffing can also result in liver damage, major brain damage, convulsions, and death. Inhalation of flammable fumes from aerosol containers frequently results in sudden death.

Marijuana. Smoking of the dried leaves and flowers of the weed *Cannabis sativa* produces feelings of euphoria. Large doses can cause hallucinations and LSD-type experiences. Marijuana goes by many names, including grass, pot, tea, and maryjane. It can be smoked, eaten, or made into tea. It is not believed to be physically addictive, but psychological dependency can occur.

Opiates. These derivatives of the opium poppy are depressants. The most common form, heroin, is a white, off-white, or brown powder known by many street names, such as "horse," "smack," or "junk." (Other opium derivatives include morphine and codeine.) Heroin can be taken orally or inhaled, although it is usually melted over a flame into a solution and injected into a vein. It causes a feeling of euphoria. The pupils dilate, and the user is likely to fall asleep. Sensory perceptions and hunger, sex, and aggressive drives are reduced.

Heroin is addictive. People become dependent at different rates, but about 20 per cent of those who experiment with heroin become addicted. Addicts suffer a number of physical and mental disorders. Loss of appetite can lead to malnutrition, and use of unsterilized needles can result in hepatitis. After a period of use, the original dose no longer provides a feeling of euphoria, and a greater amount of the drug is needed to obtain the desired results. Thus the addiction becomes increasingly expensive, and sometimes users resort to crime to support their habit.

Attempts at withdrawal result in cramps, chills, and pain. Only a small portion of addicts are ever able to permanently kick the habit. If you are searching for a new experience, heroin isn't one of the better choices you could make.

Psychedelics and Hallucinogens. The most well known of these "trip" drugs is LSD. Others in this category include mescaline, peyote, and psilocybin. These drugs, which are highly unpredictable in effect, often cause the user to perceive things that are not objectively present (hallucinate) and may result in extremes of euphoria or depression. They are not addictive, but much remains to be learned about their effects on the body.

PCP.   Also known as angel dust, goon, busy bee, crystal cyclone, and many others. Phencyclidine was developed in the late 1950s as an anesthetic for use in surgery. It was banned for use in humans when it was found to produce undesirable side effects such as agitation, hallucinations, and seizures.

PCP can be mixed with marijuana or tobacco and smoked, taken in capsule or tablet form, inhaled, or injected. In small doses there is often a feeling of euphoria at first, which is followed by depression and irritability as the effect of the drug wears off. Large doses of PCP may cause the user to appear drunk because of loss of control over speech and muscle coordination. Normally calm people may become violent and attack or even kill others or themselves. Death from PCP can thus result from the loss of coordination (people have fallen from roofs, gotten into auto accidents, drowned in shallow water), the tendency toward violent behavior, or simply from overdose of the drug itself.

Appendix C
Bibliography

CHAPTER 1   SELF-ANALYSIS

A Career Workbook for Liberal Arts Students
    Howard E. Figler
    Cranston, R. I., Carroll Press, 1975
Careers: An Overview
    Robert M. Worthington
    Englewood Cliffs, N. J., Prentice-Hall, Inc., 1977
Career Decision
    D. K. Byrn
    Washington, D. C., National Vocational Guidance Association, 1969
Career Development for the College Student
    Philip W. Dunphy (ed.)
    Cranston, R. I., Carroll Press, 1973
Career Explanation and Planning
    Bruce E. Shertzer
    Boston, Houghton Mifflin Co., 1973
Career Information Kit
    Chicago, Science Research Associates, Inc.
Career Opportunities — Community Services & Related Specialists
    Sylvia Bayliss et al. (eds.)
    Garden City, N.Y., Doubleday & Co., 1970
Career Opportunities — Marketing, Business, & Office Specialists
    Garland D. Wiggs (ed.)
    Garden City, N. Y., Doubleday — Co., 1973.
Career Perspective, Your Choice of Work
    Celia Denues
    Worthington, Ohio, Charles A. Jones Publishing Co., 1972   **159**

College Guide for Jewish Youth
 Washington, D. C., B'nai B'rith Career and Counseling Service
Concise Handbook of Occupations
 Chicago, J. G. Ferguson Publishing Co.
Decision Making in Nursing
 Jane Bailey and Karen Claus
 St. Louis, Missouri, C. V. Mosby Co., 1975
Desk Top Career Kit
 Largo, Fla., Careers, Inc.
Dictionary of Occupational Titles
 Washington, D.C., U.S. Department of Labor, Bureau of Employment Security
Dimensions of Professional Nursing
 Lucie Kelley
 New York, N.Y., Macmillan Publishing Co., 1975
Do You Want to be a Nurse
 New York, National League for Nursing
Encyclopedia of Associations, 10th ed.
 Margaret Fisk and Mary W. Pair (eds.)
 Vol. 1: National Organizations of the United States
 Vol. 2: Geographic-Executive Index
 Detroit, Gale Research Co., 1973
Encyclopedia of Business Information Sources, 3rd ed.
 Paul Wasserman (ed.)
 Detroit, Gale Research Co., 1976
Encyclopedia of Careers and Vocational Guidance
 William E. Hopke (ed.)
 Vol. I: Planning Your Career
 Vol. II: Careers and Occupations
 Garden City, N.Y., Doubleday & Co., 1975
Exploring Health Careers
 Gordon Lebowitz
 New York, N.Y., Fairchild Books & Visuals, 1973
Facts About Nursing
 Kansas City, Missouri, American Nurses' Association
Guide to Careers Through Vocational Training
 Edwin Whitfield and Richard Hoover
 New York, Robert R. Knapp, 1968
Health Careers for American Indians and Alaska Natives
 Rockville, Maryland, Indian Health Service
I Can Be Anything, Careers and Colleges for Young Women
 Joyce Slayton Mitchell
 New York, College Entrance Examination Board, 1975

If You Really Knew Me, Would You Still Like Me
    Eugene Kennedy
    Chicago, Argus Communications, 1975
Licensure to Practice Nursing
    Kansas City, Missouri, American Nurses' Association, B-17
Life Career Game
    S. S. Boocock
    Indianapolis, Ind., Bobbs-Merrill Company, Inc.
Man in a World at Work
    H. Borow
    Boston, Houghton Mifflin Co., 1964
Minority Groups in Nursing
    Kansas City, Missouri, American Nurses' Association
    Publication M-25
Modern Vocational Trends Reference Handbook
    J. Angel
    New York, World Trade Academy Press, 1963
Nature of Nursing
    Virginia Henderson
    New York, Macmillan Publishing Co., 1966
Non-Traditional Careers for Women
    Sarah Splaver
    New York, Julian Messner, 1973
Notes on Nursing: What It Is, What It Is Not
    Peter Smith
    Philadelphia, J. B. Lippincott Co., 1957
Nurses in Practice: A Perspective on Work Environment
    Marcella Davis
    St. Louis, Missouri, C. V. Mosby Co., 1975
Nursing As A Career
    Caroline Chandler and Sharon Kempf
    New York, N.Y., Dodd, Mead & Co., 1970
Nursing in Health Maintenance Organizations
    Kansas City, Missouri, American Nurses' Association, CH-7
Nursing in Society
    Josephine A. Dolan
    Philadelphia, W. B. Saunders Co., 1978
Nursing Trends
    Virginia Dryden
    Dubuque, Iowa, William C. Brown Co., 1968
Occupational Information
    Robert Hoppock
    New York, McGraw-Hill Book Co., 1976

Occupational Information
   M. F. Baer and E. C. Roeber
   Chicago, Science Research Associates, Inc., 1958
Occupational Outlook Handbook
   Washington, D. C., U. S. Department of Labor, Bureau of Labor Statistics
Orientation to Health Services
   Ruth M. Lee
   Indianapolis, Indiana, Bobbs-Merrill Educational Publishing, 1978
Patient Centered Approaches to Nursing
   Faye Abdellah
   New York, Macmillan Publishing Co., 1960
Paraprofessionals: Careers of the Future and the Present
   Sarah Splaver
   New York, Julian Messner, 1972
Pediatric Nurse Practitioners: Their Practice Today
   Kansas City, Missouri, American Nurses' Association, MC H-5
Practical Nursing Career
   New York, National League for Nursing, Pub. No. 38–1328
Preparation of Nurses for Participation in Research
   Kansas City, Missouri, American Nurses' Association, D-54
Primary Care by Nurses: Sphere of Responsibility and Accountability
   Kansas City, Missouri, American Nurses' Association, G-127, 1976
Professional Development in Psychiatric and Mental Health Nursing
   Kansas City, Missouri, American Nurses' Association, P MH-2
Quality Assurance for Nursing Care
   Kansas City, Missouri, American Nurses' Association, NS-18
Research in Nursing: Toward a Science of Health Care
   Kansas City, Missouri, American Nurses' Association
Role Conception & Vocational Success & Satisfaction: A Study of Student and Professional Nurses
   Columbus, Ohio, Ohio University Press, 1963
Scope of Practice for the Pediatric Nurse Practitioner
   Kansas City, Missouri, American Nurses' Association, MCH-7
So You Want to be a Nurse
   Alan E. Nourse and Eleanore Holliday
   New York, N.Y., Harper & Row Pubs., Inc., 1961
Steppingstones to Professional Nursing
   Kathryn Cofferty and Leone Surgarman
   St. Louis, Missouri, C. V. Mosby Co., 1971
Study of Values
   Allport, Vernon and Lindzey
   Boston, Houghton Mifflin Co., 1960
Technology — What of the Future of Nurses and Nursing
   Kansas City, Missouri, American Nurses' Association, NP-15

The Book: On the Taboo Against Knowing Who You Are
Alan Watts
New York, Random House, Vintage Books, 1972
The Challenge of Nursing
Margaret Auld and Linda Birum
St. Louis, Missouri, C. V. Mosby Co., 1974
The Dynamics of Health Care
Ruth M. French
New York, McGraw-Hill Book Co., 1974
The Expanded Role of the Nurse
New York, American Journal of Nursing, 1973
The Psychology of Careers
Donald Super
New York, Harper & Row Pubs., Inc., 1957
The Psychology of Occupations
Anne Roe
New York, John Wiley & Sons Inc., 1966
The You In Program — What's It All About
Bethesda, Maryland, DHEW, Pub. No. (NIH) 72–184
Thirteen Nurses, What They Say
Cleveland, Nursing Careers
Where Do I Go from Here With My Life
John C. Crystal and Richard N. Bolles
New York, Seabury Press, Inc., 1947
Who's Right for Nursing
New York, National Student Nurses' Association
Work Experience Handbook
William H. Pivar
San Francisco, Canfield Press, 1976
You — In Program Guide
Bethesda, Maryland, DHEW, Pub. No. (NIH) 72–188
Your Career in Nursing
Mary Searight
New York, Julian Messner, 1970
Your Future in Nursing Careers
Alice Robinson and Mary Reres
New York, Richards Rosen Press, Inc., 1975

CHAPTER 2   GOAL SETTING

A Problem Solving Approach to Nursing Care Plans
Barbara Vitale
St. Louis, Missouri, C. V. Mosby Co., 1974

Steppingstones to Professional Nursing
    Kathryn Cofferty & Leone Sugarman
    St. Louis, Missouri, C. V. Mosby Co., 1971
The Nursing Process
    Marie Seedor
    New York, Teachers College Press, 1973
Work Experience Handbook
    William H. Pivar
    San Francisco, Canfield Press, 1976

CHAPTER 3   PREPARING YOURSELF FOR SUCCESS

Beyond Success and Failure: Ways to Self-Reliance and Maturity
    Willard and Marguerite Beecher
    New York, Julian Press, Inc., 1966
I'm O.K., You're A Pain In The Neck
    Albert Vorspan
    Garden City, N. Y., Doubleday, & Co., 1976
Improving Yourself
    Gary Yanker and Jack White
    New York, Dodd, Mead & Co., 1975
Positive Addiction
    William Glasser
    New York, Harper & Row Pubs., Inc., 1976
Psycho-Cybernetics
    Maxwell Maltz
    Englewood Cliffs, N.J., Prentice-Hall, Inc., 1960
Role Conception & Vocational Success & Satisfaction: A Study of Student & Professional Nurses
    Marvin Taves
    Columbus, Ohio State University Press, 1963
Self Therapy: Techniques for Personal Growth
    Muriel Schiffman
    Menlo Park, Cal., Schiffman, 1967
The Power of Positive Thinking
    Norman Vincent Peale
    Englewood Cliffs, N. J., Prentice-Hall, Inc., 1952
The You That Could Be
    Fitzhugh Dodson
    Chicago, Follett Publishing Co., 1976
This is Earl Nightingale
    Earl Nightingale
    Garden City, N. Y., Doubleday & Co., 1969

Your Erroneous Zones
    Wayne W. Dyer
    New York, Funk & Wagnalls Co., 1976

CHAPTER 4   PLANNING YOUR CURRICULUM

Accreditation of Continuing Education in Nursing: State Nurses' Associations, National Specialty Nursing Organization, Federal Nursing Services, and State Boards of Nursing
    Kansas City, Missouri, American Nurses' Association, C OE-7
Barron's Profile of American Colleges
    Benjamin Fine
    Woodbury, N.Y., Barron's Educational Series, Inc., 1973
Choosing a College: The Test of a Person
    John C. How
    New York, Delacorte Press, 1967
College Ahead: A Guide for High School Students and Their Parents
    Eugene S. Wilson and Charles A. Bucher
    New York, Harcourt Brace Jovanovich, Inc., 1973
College Education: Key to a Professional Career in Nursing
    New York, National League for Nursing, 1972
College Proficiency Examinations and Regents External Degrees
    Albany, University of the State of New York, 1976
Continuing Education in Nursing: An Overview
    Kansas City, Missouri, American Nurses' Association, C OE-10
Dimensions of Professional Nursing
    Lucie Kelley
    New York, Macmillan Publishing Company, 1975
Educational Preparation for Nurse Practitioners and Assistants to Nurses:
    A Position Paper
    Kansas City, Missouri, American Nurses' Association, G-83
Education for Nursing: The Diploma Way
    New York, National League for Nursing, Pub. 16–1314
Guidelines for Short-Term Continuing Education Programs Preparing the
    Geriatric Nurse Practitioner
    Kansas City, Missouri, American Nurses' Association, GE-3
Guide to College Majors
    Chronicle Guidance Research Department
    Moravia, N.Y., Chronicle Guidance Publications, 1973
Guide to the Evaluation of Educational Experiences in the Armed Forces
    Washington, D.C., American Council on Education
How to Plan for College
    Frank S. Endicott
    Chicago, Rand McNally & Co., 1967

How to Prepare for College
    Abraham Lass
    New York, Washington Square Press, Inc., 1964
Licensure to Practice Nursing
    Kansas City, Missouri, American Nurses' Association, B-17
Lovejoy's College Guide, 13th ed.
    Clarence E. Lovejoy
    New York, Simon & Schuster, Inc., 1976
The Nurse as Executive
    Barbara Stevens
    Wakefield, Mass., Nursing Resources, Inc., 1975
Nurses in Practice: A Perspective on Work Environment
    Marcella Davis
    St. Louis, Missouri, C. V. Mosby Co., 1975
Pediatric Nurse Practitioners: Their Practice Today
    Kansas City, Missouri, American Nurses' Association, MCH-5
Planning for College
    Sidney Margolius
    New York, Avon Books, 1965
Practical Nursing Career
    New York, National League for Nursing, Pub. 38–1328
Preparation of Nurses for Participation in Research
    Kansas City, Missouri, American Nurses' Association, D-54
Professional Development in Psychiatric and Mental Health Nursing
    Kansas City, Missouri, American Nurses' Association, P MH-2
Recommendations on Educational Preparation and Definition of the Expanded Role and Functions of the School Nurse Practitioner
    Kansas City, Missouri, American Nurses' Association, CH-3
Research in Nursing: Toward a Science of Health Care
    Kansas City, Missouri, American Nurses' Association, D-52
Scope of Practice for the Pediatric Nurse Practitioner
    Kansas City, Missouri, American Nurses' Association, MCH-7
Standards for Continuing Education in Nursing
    Kansas City, Missouri, American Nurses' Association, COE-8
The Guide to College Life
    Joyce Slayton Mitchell
    Englewood Cliffs, N.J., Prentice-Hall, Inc., 1968
The Overeducated American
    Richard Freeman
    New York, Academic Press, Inc., 1976
The New York Times Guide to College Selection
    Ella Mazel
    New York, Quadrangle Books, 1972

Your Future in Nursing Careers
  Alice Robinson & Mary Reres
  New York, Richards Rosen Press, Inc., 1975

CHAPTER 5   HOW TO STUDY

A Guide to College Survival
  William F. Brown and Wayne H. Holtzman
  Englewood Cliffs, N. J., Prentice-Hall, Inc., 1972
A Student's Guide to Efficient Study
  D. E. James
  Elmsford, N. Y., Pergamon Press, Inc., 1967
Better Reading Book
  Elizabeth Simpson
  Chicago, Science Research Associates, Inc., 1962
Effective Reading
  Francis P. Robinson
  New York, Harper & Row Pubs., Inc., 1962
Effective Study
  Francis P. Robinson
  New York, Harper & Row Pubs., Inc., 1946
Efficient Reading
  James I. Brown
  Indianapolis, D. C. Heath & Co., 1962
Good Memory — Good Student —A Guide to Remembering What You
  Learn
  Harry Lorayne
  Nashville, Tenn., Thomas Nelson, Inc., 1972
Homework
  Grace R. Langdon and Irving W. Stout
  New York, Day, 1969
How to Become a Better Reader
  Paul Witty
  Chicago, Science Research Associates, Inc., 1953
How to Develop an Exceptional Memory
  Morris Young and Walter Gibson
  N. Hollywood, Cal., Wilshire Book Co.
How to Improve Your Memory
  James Weinland
  Scanton, Pa., Barnes & Noble Books, 1957
How to Improve Your Memory
  Dan Halacy
  New York, Watts, Franklin, Inc., 1977

How to Improve Your Memory and Concentration
    Michael Kellett
    New York, Simon & Schuster, Inc., 1975
How to Study
    Ralph C. Preston and Morton Botel
    Chicago, Science Research Associates, Inc., 1956
How to Study
    Thomas F. Staton
    New York, McQuiddy Printing Co., 1962
How to Study Better and Get Higher Marks
    Eugene H. Ehrlich
    New York, Thomas Y. Crowell Co., 1962
How to Study in College
    Walter Pauk
    Boston, Houghton Mifflin Co., 1974
I Wish I'd Known That Before I Went to College
    Judy Brown and Donald Grossfield
    New York, An Essandess Special Edition, 1966
Improving College Reading
    Lee A. Jacobus
    New York, Harcourt, Brace & World, Inc., 1967
Improving Reading Skills in College Subjects
    Marie R. Cherinton
    New York, Teachers College Press, 1961
Inhibitions of Memory Formation
    M. E. Gibbs and R. F. Mark
    New York, Plenum Publishing Corp., 1973
Key to a Better Memory
    Andrew Abbot
    Bridgeport, Ct., Vey Books
Learning to Study
    William W. Farquhar, John D. Krumboltz, and C. Gilbert Wrenn
    New York, Ronald Press Co., 1960
Man and Memory
    Daniel Halacy
    New York, Harper & Row Pubs., Inc., 1970
Memory and Attention: An Introduction to Human Information Processing
    Donald A. Norman
    New York, John Wiley & Sons, Inc., 1969
Memory: Facts & Fallacies
    I. M. Hunter
    New York, Penguin Books, Inc., 1958

Miracle of Instant Memory Power
    David Lewis
    Englewood Cliffs, N.J., Prentice-Hall, Inc., 1973
Purposeful Reading in College
    James M. McCallister
    New York, Appleton-Century-Crofts, 1942
Reading for Success in College: A Guide to Background Reading and Study Skills
    Walter Pauk
    Oshkosh, Wis., Academia Press, 1968
Reading Skills
    William D. Baker
    Englewood Cliffs, N.J., Prentice-Hall, Inc., 1953
Recall & Recognition
    J. Brown
    New York, John Wiley & Sons, Inc., 1976
Remember Anything You Want
    Virginia Krymow
    Dayton, Ohio, Arlotta Press, 1977
Remembering Made Easy
    Arthur Logan
    New York, Arco Publishing Co., Inc., 1965
Study Is Hard Work
    William H. Armstrong
    New York: Harper & Row Pubs., Inc., 1956
Study Skills: A Student's Guide for Survival
    Robert A. Carman and Royce Adams, Jr.
    New York, John Wiley & Sons, Inc., 1972
Techniques for Efficient Remembering
    Donald Laird
    New York, McGraw-Hill Book Co., 1960
The Adventure of Learning in College
    Roger H. Garrison
    New York, Harper & Row Pubs. Inc., 1954
The Art of Memory
    Francis Yates
    Chicago, University of Chicago Press, 1974
Total Recall: Enhance Your Life Through a Better Memory
    David Markoff and Denise Carcel
    New York, Grosset & Dunlap, Inc., 1976
Your Memory, How It Works & How to Improve It
    Kenneth Higbel
    Englewood Cliffs, N.J., Prentice-Hall, Inc., 1977

CHAPTER 6   HOW TO TAKE AN EXAMINATION

How to Study and Take Exams
    Lincoln Pettit
    New York, J. F. Rider, 1960
Score: The Strategy of Taking Tests
    Darrell Huff
    New York, Appleton-Century-Crofts, 1961

CHAPTER 7   HOW TO WRITE A TERM PAPER

A Manual for the Writers of Term Papers, Theses and Dissertations, 4th
    ed.
    Kate L. Turabian
    Chicago, University of Chicago Press, 1973
A Problem Solving Approach to Nursing Care Plans
    Barbara Vitale
    St. Louis, Mo., C. V. Mosby Co., 1974
A Reading Approach to College Writing
    Martha Cox
    Scranton, Pa., Chandler Publishing Co., 1971
A Research Manual for College Studies and Papers
    Cecil B. Williams
    New York, Harper & Row Pubs., Inc., 1951
Anatomy of a Theme
    Robert H. Meyer
    Beverly Hills, Cal., Glencoe Press, 1969
Books, Libraries and You: A Handbook on the Use of Reference Books
    and the Reference Resources of the Library, 3rd ed.
    Jessie Boyd et al.
    New York, Charles Scribner's Sons, 1965
Cumulative Index to Nursing and Allied Health Literature
    Glendale, Cal., Glendale Adventist Medical Center, 1977
Elements of College Writing and Reading
    P. Joseph Canoval
    New York, McGraw-Hill Book Co., 1971
Guide to the Use of Books and Libraries
    Jean Gates
    New York, McGraw-Hill Book Co., 1962
Handbook for Practical Composition
    Morriss H. Needleman
    New York, McGraw-Hill Book Co., 1968
How and Where to Look It Up
    New York, McGraw-Hill Book Co., 1958

Ideas and Patterns for Writing
 Carle B. Spotts
 New York, Holt, Rinehart and Winston, Inc., 1971
Reading, Writing, & Rhetoric, 3rd ed.
 James B. Hogins and Robert E. Yarber
 Chicago, Science Research Associates, Inc., 1975
Say It With Words
 Charles W. Ferguson
 Lincoln, University of Nebraska Press, 1954
The Experience of Writing
 William D. Baker and T. Benson Strandness
 Englewood Cliffs, N.J., Prentice-Hall, Inc., 1970
The Modern Researcher
 Jacques Barzun and Henry Graft
 New York, Harcourt, Brace & Co., 1957
The Research Paper: Gathering Library Material, Organizing and Preparing the Manuscript
 Lucyle Hooks
 Englewood Cliffs, N.J., Prentice-Hall, Inc., 1962
The Use of Books and Libraries
 Minnesota University Library School
 Minneapolis, University of Minnesota Press, 1958
The Writer's Voice: Dramatic Situations for College Writing
 Ken L. Symes
 New York, Holt, Rinehart and Winston, Inc., 1973
Using Books and Libraries
 Ella Aldrich
 Englewood Cliffs, N. J., Prentice-Hall, Inc., 1960
Writing a Technical Paper
 Donald H. Menzel and Howard M. Jones
 New York, McGraw-Hill Book Co., 1961
Writing: Process and Product
 Susan Miller
 Cambridge, Mass., Winthrop Publishers, Inc., 1976
Writing Without Teachers
 Peter Elbow
 New York, Oxford University Press, 1973

CHAPTER 8 FINANCING YOUR EDUCATION

A Parent's Guide to College Planning
 Frank S. Endicott
 New York, Rand McNally & Co., 1967

Anyone Can Get into College
 Herbert B. Livesey
 New York, Viking Press, Inc., 1971
Borrowing for College: A Guide for Students and Parents
 Washington, D. C., United States Office of Education
College Scholarship Guide
 Clarence E. Lovejoy and Theodore Jones
 New York, Simon & Schuster, Inc.
Complete Planning for College: The Kiplinger Guide to Your Education
 Beyond High School
 New York, McGraw-Hill Book Co., 1962
Financial Assistance for College Students: Undergraduates
 Washington, D. C., United States Office of Education
Financial Information National Directory
 Chicago, American Medical Association, 1972
Going Right On
 Princeton, N.J., College Entrance Examination Board
Health Careers for American Indians and Alaska Natives
 Rockville, Maryland, Indian Health Service
How About College Financing? A Guide for Parents and College-Bound
 Students
 Norman S. Feingold
 Washington, D. C., American School Counselor Association
How to Beat the High Cost of College
 Claire Cox
 New York, Dial Press, 1971
How to Get Money for College
 Benjamin Fine and Sidney Eisenberg
 New York, Doubleday & Co., 1964
I Wish I'd Known That Before I Went to College
 Judy Brown and Donald Grossfield
 New York, An Essandess Special Edition, 1966
Need A Lift
 Indianapolis, American Legion Education and Scholarship Program,
 Americanism and Children and Youth Division
Planning for College
 Sidney Margolius
 New York, Avon Books, 1965
Scholarships and Loans for Beginning Education in Nursing
 New York, National League for Nursing, Pub. 41–410
Scholarships for American Indians
 Albuquerque, Bureau of Indian Affairs
Student Financial Help: A Guide to Money for College
 Louis T. and Joyce W. Scaring
 Garden City, N. Y., Doubleday & Co., 1974

Your College Education: How to Pay for It
    Sarah Splaver
    New York, Julian Messner, 1964

CHAPTER 9   ADJUSTMENT TO THE COLLEGE ENVIRONMENT

A Guide to College Survival
    William F. Brown and Wayne H. Holtzman
    Englewood Cliffs, N. J., Prentice-Hall, Inc., 1972
Beyond Success and Failure: Ways to Self-Reliance and Maturity
    Willard and Marguerite Beecher
    New York, Pocket Books, Inc., 1971
Body Language and the Social Order
    Albert Scheflen
    Englewood Cliffs, N.J., Prentice-Hall, Inc., 1973
Communication for Nurses
    Florence Lockerby
    St. Louis, Missouri, C. V. Mosby Co., 1956
Communication in Nursing
    Thora Kron
    Philadelphia, W. B. Saunders Co., 1967
Getting the Most Out of College
    Margaret Bennett, Molly Lewin, and Dorothy McKay
    New York, McGraw-Hill Book Co., 1957
How to Do a University
    Andrew Barclay, William Crano, Charles Thornton, and Arnold
        Werner
    New York, John Wiley & Sons, Inc., 1971
How to Talk with People
    Irving J. Lee
    New York, Harper & Row Pubs., Inc., 1952
Husband/Father/Humanitarian/Specialist/Nurse
    New York, National League for Nursing
I Wish I'd Known That Before I Went to College
    Judy Brown and Donald Grossfield
    New York, An Essandess Special Edition, 1966
Interacting with Patients
    Kenneth H. Larson and Joyce S. Hays
    New York, Macmillan Publishing Co., 1963
Interpersonal Relations in Nursing
    Hildegard Peplau
    New York, G. P. Putnam's Sons, 1952
Introduction to College
    Bert D. Anderson
    New York, Holt, Rinehart and Winston, Inc., 1969

Love and Sex in Plain Language
    Eric W. Johnson
    Philadelphia, J. B. Lippincott Co., 1965
Love and the Facts of Life
    Evelyn M. Duvall
    New York, Association Press, 1963
Love, Sex and the Teenager
    Rhoda Lorand
    Riverside, N.J., Macmillan Publishing Co., 1965
Mastering the College Challenge
    Bette Soldwedel
    Riverside, N. J., Macmillan Publishing Co., 1965
Messages of the Body
    John Spiegel and Paul Machotka
    New York, Free Press, 1974
Motivation and Personality
    Abraham Maslow
    New York, Harper & Row Pub., Inc., 1954
Nonverbal Communication
    Jurgen Ruesch and Weldon Kees
    Berkeley, University of California Press, 1956
Body Language
    Julius Fast
    New York, M. Evans & Co., 1970
Nonverbal Communication: Readings with Commentary
    Shirley Weitz
    New York, Oxford University Press, 1974
Nonverbal Communication with Patients: Back to the Human Touch
    New York, John Wiley & Sons, Inc., 1977
Nurse Patient Communication
    Garland Lewis
    Dubuque, Iowa, William C. Brown Co., Pubs., 1973
On Becoming an Educated Person, 4th ed.
    Virginia Voeks
    Philadelphia, W. B. Saunders Co., 1979
Patients Are People
    Minna Filed
    New York, Columbia University Press, 1967
Patient Centered Approaches to Nursing
    Faye Abdellah
    New York, Macmillan Publishing Co., 1960
Planning Patient Care
    Lucile Lewis
    Dubuque, Iowa, William C. Brown Co., Pubs., 1970

Psychology of Personal and Social Adjustment
    Henry Clay Lindgren
    New York, American Book Co., 1959
The Allied Health Professional and the Patient
    Ruth Purtilo
    Philadelphia, W. B. Saunders Co., 1974
The Art and Skill of Getting Along with People
    Sylvanus M. Duval
    Englewood Cliffs, N. J., Prentice-Hall, Inc., 1961
The College Drug Scene
    James T. Carey
    Englewood Cliffs, N.J., Prentice-Hall, Inc., 1968
The College Scene: Students Tell It Like It Is
    James A. Foley and Robert K. Foley
    New York, Cowles, 1969
The Communication of Emotional Meaning
    Joel R. Davitz, et al.
    New York, McGraw-Hill Book Co., 1964
Forgotten Language
    Erich Fromm
    New York, Holt, Rinehart & Winston, 1951
The Patient as a Person
    Paul Ramsey
    New Haven, Yale University Press, 1970
The Psychology of College Success: A Dynamic Approach
    Henry Clay Lindren
    New York, American Book Co., 1969
What About Teenage Marriage
    Jeanne Sakol
    New York, Julian Messner, 1961
Working with Others for Patient Care
    Grace Peterson
    Dubuque, Iowa, William C. Brown Co., Pubs., 1973

CHAPTER 10   **EMPLOYMENT DURING AND AFTER COLLEGE**

Dun & Bradstreet Directories
    N.Y., Dun & Bradstreet
Encyclopedia of Associations, 10th ed.
    Margaret Fisk and Mary W. Pair (eds.)
    Detroit, Gale Research Co., 1976
Encyclopedia of Business Information Sources, 3rd ed.
    Paul Wasserman (ed.)
    Detroit, Mich., Gale Research Co., 1976

Go Hire Yourself an Employer
    Richard Irish
    Garden City, N.Y., Anchor Books, 1973
Moody's Industrials
    New York, Moody's Investor Service Inc.
On-The-Job Training and Where to Get It
    Robert Liston
    New York, Julian Messner, 1973
Summer Employment Directory of the United States, 26th rev. ed.
    Mypena A. Leith
    Cincinnati, National Directory Service, Inc., 1976
The National Directory of Employment Services
    Detroit, Mich., Gale Research Co.
Thomas Register
    New York, Thomas Publishing Co.
Work Experience Handbook
    William H. Pivar
    San Francisco, Canfield Press, 1976

Index